Caregiver Stress and
Staff Support in Illness,
Dying, and Bereavement

Caregiver Stress and Staff Support in Illness, Dying, and Bereavement

Edited by

Irene Renzenbrink

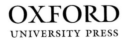

OXFORD
UNIVERSITY PRESS

OXFORD

UNIVERSITY PRESS

Great Clarendon Street, Oxford OX2 6DP

Oxford University Press is a department of the University of Oxford.
It furthers the University's objective of excellence in research, scholarship,
and education by publishing worldwide in

Oxford   New York

Auckland   Cape Town   Dar es Salaam   Hong Kong   Karachi
Kuala Lumpur   Madrid   Melbourne   Mexico City   Nairobi
New Delhi   Shanghai   Taipei   Toronto

With offices in

Argentina   Austria   Brazil   Chile   Czech Republic   France   Greece
Guatemala   Hungary   Italy   Japan   Poland   Portugal   Singapore
South Korea   Switzerland   Thailand   Turkey   Ukraine   Vietnam

Oxford is a registered trade mark of Oxford University Press
in the UK and in certain other countries

Published in the United States
by Oxford University Press Inc., New York

British Library Cataloguing in Publication Data

Data available

Library of Congress Cataloging in Publication Data

Library of Congress Control Number: 2010942949

Typeset in Minion by Glyph International Bangalore, India
Printed in Great Britain
on acid-free paper by
CPI Antony Rowe, Chippenham, Wiltshire

ISBN 978–0–19–959040–7

10 9 8 7 6 5 4 3 2 1

To my mother, Aafje A. Heineke-Sieuwerts,
my first teacher in caring

Acknowledgements

I offer my sincere thanks to all the contributors who devoted precious time and energy to this combined effort. I am also very grateful to Nicola Wilson and Jenny Wright at Oxford University Press for their guidance and support. I would like to acknowledge my mentor and colleague, Sandra Bertman, who, in her inimitable and creative way, kindly wrote the Foreword. I also need to acknowledge the influence of Robert Fulton, David Oliviere, Colin Murray Parkes, Phyllis Silverman, and Joan Berzoff, and finally the late Peter Marris, on my professional development and my writing. Dr Roger Buckle provided the holding environment that enabled me to thrive in some very challenging workplaces, and my partner, Rudie Heineke, has given me the unconditional love, support, and encouragement that I need to thrive in everything I do.

Foreword

Dr Sandra Bertman

There's an old Handelsman cartoon: Two men are seated, drinking at the bar. One says to the other, 'Strange, isn't it. Usually I'm a very caring person. But in your case, for some reason, I don't give a damn'.

Not giving a damn in our work with the dying and bereaved, or with our colleagues, is an anathema. Most of us have chosen these professions because we do care and want our caring to make a difference to our patients, clients, and colleagues.

The essence of our work is lending presence, accepting silence, and being willing to enter into another's suffering, so the other's story is able to unfold, be voiced, and acknowledged. This 'exquisite witness', defined by the wise, soft-spoken therapist and author, Shep Jeffers, is one who 'observes more than acts, listens more than talks, and follows more than leads'.

We are often reminded that our resources for compassion are finite; in order to be continually attuned to others' distress, our own batteries need recharging. Ennui, boredom, lack of interest, even indifference are evidence of apathy, what the American newspaper editor Horace Greenley defines as 'a sort of living oblivion'. Attention must be paid to self-care. A recent *New York Times* review of Oren Harman's *The Price of Altruism* opens with an allusion to the familiar safety message prior to the take-off of every flight, 'secure your own oxygen mask before assisting anyone else'.

Complexities and uncertainties are inherent in all therapeutic relationships. Sometimes we just can't seem to care. What are the 'some reason[s]', as in the cartoon, 'for not giv[ing] a damn'? Burnout? Compassion fatigue? Work overload? Grief overload? Staff dissension? Personal frustrations and distractions? Feelings of inadequacy and helplessness? How do we sustain enough sympathy, patience, and love to recycle it again and again, especially when we know the relationship might end shortly or abruptly? This book is comprehensive, even encyclopaedic, in identifying the multitude of stressors that can affect the ability to maintain compassionate involvement.

Various clinicians believe that the seeds of healing lie dormant within our own beings (be we counsellor or client), able to break through and bloom. Some remind us to be gentle with ourselves. We are only human beings, as the Turkish proverb puts it: 'harder than iron, stronger than stone, and more fragile than a rose'. Exercising sensitive timing, one might appropriately steer the conversation to refocus on one's strengths and possibilities rather than solely on the negatives—what one can't do or isn't doing.

In this age of evidence-based practice, documented, up-to-date research on caregiver stress and staff support is absolutely necessary for practitioners and educators in today's world of healthcare. This book acknowledges the early pioneers; it builds on their work and equips the reader with the most recent studies of experts in the field. Yet this compendium offers much more. I'm reminded of the sign that Albert Einstein allegedly kept on his wall: 'Not everything that counts can be counted and not everything that can be counted counts'. We are privy to ample anecdotal revelatory accounts of the personal vulnerabilities, strains, doubts, mishaps, mistakes, and failures—as well as the creative approaches of our colleagues which not only inform the research, demonstrate resilience, and the ability to persevere when things go awry; but ultimately infuse this book with an unexpected and refreshing credibility.

Three themes weave themselves through the chapters: compassion, connection, and collaboration, and the pendulum seems to be swinging to a new professionalism. Whether caregiver and patient, or caregiver and supervisor, connection and collaboration has clearly moved from the paternalistic to the patient-centred, and, even more so, to a relationship-centred ideal. Physician Rachel Naomi Remen, cited often throughout this book, speaks adamantly of our role as neither fixer nor helper, but as one of service. She defines this relationship as one between equals—the wholeness in one serving the wholeness in the other. Paradoxically, rather than being depleting, our work is refuelling. As the saying goes, 'A candle loses none of its light by lighting another candle'. Drawing on their own experiences, the authors concur that a capacity for empathy and compassionate involvement prevents rather than causes burnout. The meeting of two personalities often creates its own invigorating synergy.

This book resonates with the intensity and energy of its editor. In every chapter, the reader feels the reverberations of Renzenbrink's concept of 'relentless self-care'. Her contributors were chosen for their honesty and courage in engaging in reflective practice rather than solely for their quantitative modes of thorough and excellent research.

The poet Emily Dickinson reminds us 'The possible's slow fuse is lit by imagination'. This compendium gives us all the tools—research, philosophical insights, soul-searching personal accounts, poetry, and practical techniques. Let its bountiful generative sparks challenge, support, and revitalize us in our chosen work.

Contents

List of contributors

Rena Arshinoff
Rabbi and Chaplain,
University Health Network,
Toronto Western Hospital Division,
Toronto, Ontario, Canada

Sandra Bertman
Distinguished Professor,
Thanatology and Arts,
Mt. Ida College,
Newton, Massachusetts, USA

Ted Bowman
Family and Grief Educator,
Consultant and Author,
St Paul, Minnesota, USA

Susan Breiddal
Counsellor, Palliative Response Team,
Victoria Hospice Society,
Victoria, BC, Canada

Amy Yin Man Chow
Assistant Professor,
Department of Social Work and
Social Administration,
The University of Hong Kong,
Hong Kong

Andrea Dechamps
Director of Social Work, Bereavement
and Welfare,
St Christopher's Hospice,
Sydenham, London, UK

Rosemary Feeley
Social Worker/Family Therapist,
Victoria, Australia

Pam Firth
Deputy Director
Isabel Hospice,
Hertfordshire, UK

Michael Kearney
Palliative Medicine and Hospice
Physician,
Santa Barbara,
California, USA

William Lamers
Psychiatrist and Hospice
Physician,
The Lamers Medical Group,
California, USA

Philip Larkin
Professor of Clinical Nursing
(Palliative Care),
University College, Dublin, and
Our Lady's Hospice and
Care Services,
Harold's Cross,
Dublin, Ireland

Val Maasdorp
Clinical Director,
Island Hospice,
Harare, Zimbabwe

Yvonne Yi Wood Mak
Medical Officer, Bradbury Hospice,
Palliative Care/Oncology Unit,
Pamela Youde Nethersole Eastern
Hospital,
Hong Kong

Danny Nugus
Service Development and
Training Manager,
Winston's Wish,
Gloucestershire, UK

Irene Renzenbrink
Social Worker and Art Therapist,
Lakeside Education and Training,
Australia and Canada

Ann Saville
Social Worker,
Peninsula Health,
Victoria, Australia

Neil Thompson
Director,
Avenue Consulting,
Wrexham, Wales, UK

Mary Vachon
Professor, Department of Psychiatry
and Dalla Lana School of Public Health,
University of Toronto,
Toronto, Canada

Wendy Wainwright
Manager, Psychosocial Services,
Victoria Hospice Society
Victoria, BC, Canada

Radhule Weininger
Clinical Psychologist,
Santa Barbara,
California, USA

Robin Youngson
Anaesthetic Specialist,
Waitemata District Health Board,
Auckland, New Zealand

Introduction

Irene Renzenbrink

In a workshop I conducted on the topic of burnout and compassion fatigue several years ago I asked a group of palliative care professionals to list some of their self-care activities. One of the workshop participants wrote the following: 'walking the dog, running, clinical supervision, healthy food, holidays, good relationships, sleep, therapy, crying/shouting, art/writing, gallows humour, drinking and cultural activities'. It was an interesting mix of physical, psychological, and social activities that were being used to promote well being. However, most participants also emphasized the importance of working in a well-managed organization that recognized and valued their efforts. Schaufeli (1999, p. 30) suggests that burnout is a result of a lack of reciprocity at an interpersonal level, and withdrawal from the organization is the result of lack of reciprocity at an organizational level. It seems that a balance between 'investments and outcomes' is crucial. As Schaufeli puts it, 'it is not just about working too long and too hard with difficult recipients'. Having once worked for a service where the head of the organization engaged in a 'divide and rule' management style using bullying and favouritism, I can testify to the fact that reciprocity can easily be corroded when an employee's investment is no longer proportionate to the gains.

If I were to list some of the themes that might be relevant to a consideration of Caregiver Stress and Staff Support in Illness, Dying, and Bereavement, they would include an understanding of stress, resilience, and coping; transference and countertransference; burnout, compassion fatigue, and vicarious traumatization; management practices; teamwork; clinical supervision and peer support; moral distress; models of grief and loss as well as social and organizational theory. All of these perspectives, and more, are represented in this book and serve to illustrate the complexity of the subject. We have come a long way from the days when individual counselling, staff support groups, or a long vacation were considered to be an antidote to stress in the workplace.

My interest in caregiver stress and staff support began over almost 40 years ago when, as a new social work graduate, I was literally thrown in the deep end of a large teaching hospital. As I have described elsewhere (Renzenbrink, 2004), I'd been assigned to the cancer ward and my job was to 'place' dying patients in nursing homes. Although I had worked in hospitals during my student years the difference was that I now had a distinct professional role and responsibility to relieve the patients' suffering, at least from a psychosocial perspective. Although I was offered supervision I did not feel that I could express my true feelings with my superior, and when I did confide in her, was immediately offered an appointment with one of the hospital psychiatrists. The message was clear. I was the one with the problem and my only alternative was to leave.

Up until that time I had no knowledge of the modern hospice movement, but in 1977 an Australian nurse, Sr. Katherine Kingsbury, was awarded a Winston Churchill Fellowship to investigate 'models of domiciliary care for the frail aged, the handicapped and the dying'. Katherine visited St Christopher's Hospice in London, UK, the Royal Victoria Hospital in Montreal, Canada, and the Hospice of New Haven in Connecticut, USA. Her findings and subsequent report formed the foundation for the Australian hospice movement. Since I was working in a paediatric oncology unit at that time, Katherine and I had many conversations about the care of dying children as well as the impact of the work. I was then invited to join the steering committee which led to the establishment of the first hospice home care programme in Australia. After reading Sandol Stoddard's book, *The Hospice Movement: A Better Way of Caring for the Dying* (1978), I was particularly impressed with the attention that was given to the needs of staff. It was Dame Cicely Saunders, founder of St Christopher's Hospice, who said,

> We in this work are somehow missing an outer layer of skin and must take care to renew ourselves.

Dr Elisabeth Kübler Ross, whose pioneering work throughout the world did so much to raise the consciousness about death and dying in the 1970s, also emphasized the need for staff to receive support, and in particular, to become aware of their own history of loss and 'unfinished business' so that they could be truly available to their patients.

It was in Kingsbury's book, based on her Churchill Fellowship report, *I Want to Die at Home* (1978), that I was first introduced to Mary Vachon's writing about staff stress and staff support, and I am particularly grateful to Mary for agreeing to review her distinguished involvement in the field of palliative care and to share key research findings and practice wisdom about occupational stress. It is entirely appropriate that her chapter is the first in this book.

While my first social work position had already awakened an interest in the care of caregivers, my commitment to promoting the issue was firmly reinforced by all my subsequent experiences. In the 1980s I worked for a funeral company to establish a bereavement support services division. On my first day at work I was greeted with the news that the father of a boy whose funeral was being arranged had committed suicide and there was to be a double funeral. I was asked to 'support' the family. One of the greatest sources of stress as a professional caregiver is the feeling of impotence and inadequacy in the face of tragedy and suffering when our altruistic impulse and our professional training urges us to help. My understanding of what is helpful and unhelpful when caregivers experience grief and stress was further informed by my involvement in the self-help movement and in the area of traumatic bereavement and disaster recovery following shooting incidents in Australia and New Zealand in the late 1980s and early 1990s. I clearly remember the cry of frustration from a minister in a disaster-affected community when he was besieged by well-meaning mental health professionals. In his words, 'If anyone else offers to debrief me, I'll take my bloody trousers off.' (Renzenbrink, 2004).

In today's world of advanced communication technology where we are exposed to all kinds of suffering on a daily basis and where, as one of our authors, Radhule

Weininger, puts it so eloquently, 'fear is seeping in through the cracks of our social and political fabric', we are more than ever in danger of compassion overload and fatigue. A patient education pamphlet on stress management produced in 2004 by the Mayo Clinic refers to 'techno-stress', the stress caused by cell phones, laptop or palm sized computers, email, voicemail, and pagers which allow us to be available at almost any time (p. 3). When a colleague returned to work after a period of sick leave he found 1,000 emails in his inbox; and in an article about her working day, Christine Murray (2010), Bereavement Coordinator at St Christopher's Hospice, writes that choosing when to look at her emails is part of her own self-care. Muller (2010, p. 5) sums up some of these pressures when he says, 'In a world gone mad with speed, potential and choice, we continually overestimate what we can do, build, fix, care for, or make happen in one day'.

Another layer of stress that we need to consider arises from the awareness of the world's pain in addition to our already complex family, social, and working lives, and the rapid pace of life. We know so much more about disaster and strife in other places than our own, and television, radio, and the internet bring it all home to us literally but without corresponding opportunities to act, or to absorb these events in a meaningful way. How to respond to others in compassionate and helpful ways but without going under ourselves is not always clear, and this is a challenge that many of the authors in this book address.

Fortunately there are signs of change at a systemic level. There is new evidence of many healthcare reforms which aim to foster greater compassion in working with severely ill or injured people or which address the needs of the bereaved in the workplace. Having attended a 'Schwartz Round' at Massachusetts General Hospital while participating in an international social work exchange programme in 2000, I was impressed by the honesty of both patients and doctors and the attempts to bridge the traditional gulf between them. The focus of the round that I attended was on the topic of seeking a second opinion when a patient has been diagnosed with a terminal condition. In this case the treating doctor expressed his dismay about 'his' patient's apparent lack of confidence in him, while the patient explained that he felt the need to leave no stone unturned in his fight for life. The Schwartz Center was established in 1995 by the family of Kenneth Schwartz, who died of lung cancer at age 40. The Center aims to educate and support caregivers in the art of compassionate healthcare and its success has been demonstrated through rigorous evaluation and research.

As the author and powerful advocate for the Charter for Compassion, British religious affairs commentator Karen Armstrong (2009) takes the challenge far beyond healthcare alone. A former Roman Catholic nun, Armstrong has harnessed the wisdom of worldwide religious traditions to promote compassion throughout organizations and communities everywhere. Hopeful of broad social change, Armstrong remains realistic when she says, 'I don't expect the whole world will fall into each other's arms. This is the beginning of a long process. I see it as re-educating people in the concept of compassion. Most people are not aware that it is at the centre of the world's faiths' (p. A15).

Several years ago I was approached by an organization providing case management for clients with severe disabilities to conduct a workshop about stress management.

The manager who contacted me was proud of a new slogan that he and his colleagues had created, 'We do *even* more with less'. I pointed out that not only were they asking staff to do more in a climate of diminished resources, but *even* more, and wondered about the wisdom of such a message when staff were already working long hours without additional pay.

In Chapter 2 Neil Thompson discusses work place well being from a psychosocial perspective and analyses key issues and leadership responsibilities related to stress recognition and management, emphasizing the need for an approach which acknowledges yet goes beyond individual psychology. He argues that social and organizational factors need to be considered and that organizational factors need to encompass strategic as well as operational concerns.

In Chapter 3, Robin Youngson describes his efforts and motivation for establishing a Centre for Compassion in Healthcare in Auckland, New Zealand. Inspired by a personal experience when his daughter was severely injured and treated in the hospital where Robin worked as an anaesthetic specialist, Robin is currently engaged in a worldwide campaign to promote greater compassion in healthcare.

In Chapter 4, Radhule Weinger and Michael Kearney explore the prevention of compassion fatigue through the development of Exquisite Empathy in clinical practice. Their unique approach to medical education and supervision is heavily influenced by Buddhist psychology and Mindfulness Meditation. With many years of experience in both medicine and psychotherapy these gifted and sensitive practitioners address the challenge of finding a balance 'between caring for ourselves and being open to the world we encounter'. It is argued that ironically, compassionate and closer empathic involvement is less likely to cause burnout and compassion fatigue than the other way around.

Yvonne Yi Wood Mak, from Hong Kong, provides a unique view of the hospice doctor's experience from both a professional perspective and from her own experience as a cancer patient in Chapter 5. She suggests that 'attending to our being' is a form of self-care and that reflective practice can transform our stresses into strengths. It is a thoughtful account that demonstrates the link between the quality of professional work and the personal development and growth of the caregiver.

A further exploration of the impact of a staff member's illness on a team caring for the dying is the subject of Chapter 6, contributed by hospice social workers Ann Saville and Rosemary Feeley from Australia. These two experienced professionals highlight the value of a more open and honest approach to working in a setting where the careful merging of professional and personal boundaries involves taking some risks. They describe the kind of management and leadership style that promotes wellbeing in the whole team when a team member is faced with a personal crisis.

In developing the proposal for this book I felt strongly that personal reflections by professional caregivers should be included because, as Moon would say, 'aspects of work, love and life complement and enhance one another' (2002, p. 34). In healthcare settings where emotional intensity and human suffering is witnessed on a daily basis it is difficult if not impossible to control or limit emotional involvement. During my social work training we were told to practise 'detached concern'. Moon suggests that feminist psychology has challenged traditional polarization of the personal and the professional. After all, the capacity to form close attachments and to nurture others pervades many aspects of our lives and is not only confined to our assigned professional roles. Professionals will also have their own share of personal experiences of illness, crisis, and loss to contend with, and will be called on to respond with empathy and compassion in other areas of life.

Chapter 7, in which Val Maasdorp describes some of the extraordinary pressures faced by the staff at Island Hospice in Harare, Zimbabwe, provides an inspiring account of how staff cope with stress in a country beset with the greatest of economic and political pressures. Despite what some might consider to be insurmountable obstacles, there remains a core of resilience, optimism and good humour amongst the staff.

Against a background of powerful taboos surrounding death and bereavement amongst the Chinese population in Hong Kong, Amy Yin Man Chow describes Project ENABLE in Chapter 8. An educational programme designed to develop greater competence in professionals who care for the dying and bereaved, this approach has been shown to reduce death anxiety, enhance self care and personal relationships as well as provide better service to clients.

An example of an enlightened and creative management approach in a hospice programme is offered in Chapter 9 and provides not only the perspective of a leader and manager, Wendy Wainwright, but also that of a member of the counselling team, Susan Breiddal. Susan provides a lively, scrupulously honest, and at times, poetic account of the daily challenges in finding a healthy and happy work/life balance.

In a similar vein Andrea Dechamps (Chapter 10) provides an imaginative and thoughtful analysis of management and leadership issues at St Christopher's Hospice in the UK, where she leads a large team of social workers. She argues that leaders and their teams need a commitment to reflection and dialogue in a work culture that is open to self-care and self-awareness. Andrea also addresses the challenge of balancing performance expectations with the emotional needs of staff in a climate of reduced healthcare budgets.

In Chapter 11, Danny Nugus, a social worker and team leader at the children's bereavement support service Winston's Wish, presents a unique model for working with bereaved children, again creatively balancing the needs of staff with professional responsibilities for clients. He extrapolates from the needs of bereaved children to the needs of staff and suggests ways in which staff can use their understanding of loss and bereavement to develop more resilience in relation to their work.

Philip Larkin (Chapter 12), a Professor of Nursing in Dublin, examines the challenges facing nurses and other health care professionals at a time of global economic crisis and, in particular, reduced health care budgets in Ireland. Stressors related to staff shortages and a lack of resources can affect staff well being and the ability to maintain compassionate involvement. He speaks of the need to 'balance the science and artistry' of nursing by drawing on 'inner wisdom' and also explores the meaning of compassion which he feels is still ill-defined and under-researched in palliative care.

The value of clinical supervision in maintaining quality service for clients but also in promoting well being in professional caregivers is the focus of Pam Firth's chapter (Chapter 13). Pam reviews recent research into the efficacy of supervision and how it might be offered in different settings for different professional groups. She describes a model she herself has developed in the hospice where she provides leadership and support to a wide range of staff.

Chapter 14 is based on Rena Arshinoff's experience as a nurse, Rabbi and hospital chaplain and offers the concept of spiritual care as a tool for healing. While the main focus of Rena's chapter is on nurses, her suggestion "that the provision of spiritual care offers a key contribution to healing, connection and self growth and permits sharing in the community and the recognition of the holiness of life" has relevance for all caregivers.

'Reflections on caring: A brief essay on presence' is the title of Ted Bowman's chapter (Chapter 15) and is based on Ted's extensive experience in education, training and counselling. As Ted himself explains, it is a chapter which 'utilizes the twin filters of poetry therapy or bibliotherapy as well as the framework of the ethical-spiritual will'. It is a fitting chapter to end on before American hospice pioneer William (Bill) Lamers provides his remarkable insights into the issues faced by caregivers in the Afterword.

From my earliest experiences of professional life as a social worker I have been convinced of the importance of staff support, not only to ensure the highest quality of care for patients and clients, but also for maintaining well being and morale in caregivers. As Mary Vachon observes at the end of Chapter One, 'There is no doubt that in some ways care has improved, in other ways care needs to continue to be improved ... it is not a time to be complacent'.

I hope that this collection of insights, reflections, practice examples and research findings from a highly experienced and talented group of professionals from various disciplines and several countries will encourage readers to stay alert and alive in their work and to keep searching for improvements in the care of caregivers.

References

Armstrong, K. (2009). The global case for compassion. Article in *Vancouver Sun*, 25 September 2009.

Kingsbury, K. (1978). *I Want to Die at Home*. Melbourne: Fraser and Jenkinson.

Muller, W. (2010). *A Life of Being, Having, and Doing Enough*. New York: Harmony Books.

Murray, C. (2010). Day in the life End of life care. *Therapy Today*, April.

Renzenbrink, I. (2004). Relentless self care. In P. Silverman and J. Berzoff (2004). *Living with Dying: A Handbook for End of Life Care Practitioners*. New York: Columbia University Press.

Schaufeli, W. (1999). Burnout. In J. Firth-Cozens and R. Payne (eds), *Stress in Health Professionals*. Chichester: John Wiley and Sons.

Stoddard, S. (1978). *The Hospice Movement: A Better Way of Caring for the Dying*. New York: Vintage.

Stress Management, Mayo Foundation for Education and Research Publication, 2004.

Chapter 1

Four decades of selected research in hospice/palliative care: have the stressors changed?

Mary L.S. Vachon

Since the early 1970s I have been involved in researching, studying, writing, and lecturing about the subject of occupational stress in oncology, hospice, and palliative care. This chapter will set the context for the emergence of the hospice/palliative care movement and review the research on the topic of occupational stress, reflecting on the similarities and differences in the field over time with regard to research findings, concepts and frameworks for understanding the subject, as well as some current approaches to understanding individual differences in coping and response to stress. This chapter will draw liberally on several previous publications.

Setting the context: the early days

The modern hospice movement dates back to the development of St Christopher's Hospice in 1967. In North America the movement began in 1974 in the United States with the opening of the Connecticut Hospice (initially a home care programme) and in Canada with the Saint Boniface Terminal Care Unit in Winnipeg, Manitoba, and the Royal Victoria Hospital Palliative Care Unit in Montreal, Quebec (Vachon, 1999).

Prior to the emergence of the hospice movement there was a small literature on the care of the dying and their caregivers written by such pioneers as Feifel (1950), Folta (1965), Fox (1959), Fulton (1965), Glaser and Strauss (1964, 1965, 1968), Hinton (1967), Quint (later Benoliel) (1966, 1967), Saunders (1959), and Sudnow (1967). Kübler-Ross's landmark book *On Death and Dying* (1969) had appeared, and across North America patients were being expected to go through the five prescribed stages of death and dying (Vachon, 1999). Some interventions had begun to help staff care for the dying persons with whom they were working (Artiss and Levine, 1973; Klagsbrun, 1970; from Vachon, 1999).

Personal involvement

At a personal level, during my childhood I had many experiences with family deaths which predisposed me to be interested in how families and professionals cope with death and tragedy.

During my last year of my diploma in nursing at the Massachusetts General Hospital (MGH), I heard a lecture on grief by Dr Tom Hackett, describing the theories about grief that had emerged from the Cocoanut Grove fire (Lindemann, 1944). I was able to immediately apply the concepts of this lecture to a patient and made my decision to go into psychiatric nursing, in order to be able to learn how to talk with patients. Early in my career I learned that the presenting problem of the patient was only part of the picture. I also became aware that as caregivers we needed to listen with the 'third ear' to hear the patient's real story.

In 1969 my husband and I moved to Toronto. My professional involvement in the area of occupational stress came when I asked the psychiatrist with whom I was working, Dr Stan Freeman, at the Clarke Institute of Psychiatry in Toronto, what I could do to help a young woman I had met through church deal with the fact that the melanoma diagnosed during her pregnancy with her fourth child had recurred and her life expectancy was limited. Dr Freeman said that he didn't know, but if I was interested in such issues there had been a request from Princess Margaret Hospital (PMH), a world-renowned cancer hospital, for psychiatrists to work with the nurses about their feelings about dying patients. I was invited to join my colleagues, Drs Alan Lyall and Patricia Nestor, and we went to PMH.

I was a member of the Department of Social and Community Psychiatry at the Clarke. We were mandated to do research into primary, secondary, and tertiary prevention using the work of Dr Gerald Caplan (1964). We undertook to investigate the stress of staff working with cancer patients and to develop programmes of intervention for staff members. Our agreement was that we would be able to assess the efficacy of the work we were doing (Rochester, Vachon, and Lyall, 1974; Vachon, 1976, 1978; Vachon, Lyall, and Freeman, 1978). The work at Princess Margaret led to other studies of intervention with women with breast cancer and with newly bereaved women (Vachon, Lyall, Rogers, et al., 1980, 1981–2).

In these early days in the field, caregivers of many disciplines involved in the care of the dying and bereaved had begun to meet and present research findings through organizations such as the Foundation of Thanatology at Columbia University, New York, under the leadership of Dr Austin Kutscher. My introduction to the hospice/palliative care movement began one day in 1974 when Dr Lyall returned from a medical meeting saying that he had met a young urologist, Dr Balfour Mount, who had a vision of opening a unit at the Royal Victoria Hospital in Montreal to care for the terminally ill. The unit was to be based in part on Dr Cicely Saunders' work at St Christopher's Hospice.

Quebec is primarily a French-speaking province. The word 'hospice' translates to 'poor house' in French, so Dr Mount looked for a new term and developed the concept of a 'palliative care' unit. To palliate is to 'alleviate (disease) without curing' (Health and Welfare Canada, 1981, p. 1). Dr Lyall suggested to Dr Mount that since our team had already studied the stress of staff at Princess Margaret Hospital we might study the stress of the staff of the newly developing Royal Victoria Hospital palliative care unit (Vachon, 1999, p. 230).

Dr Mount also suggested that we attend an upcoming meeting in 1974 organized by Dr John Fryer and Ken Spillman of the Philadelphia Ars Moriendi group. This meeting led to the development of the International Work Group on Death, Dying, and Bereavement (IWG). This meeting was attended by leaders from around the world.

Dr Cicely Saunders spoke about St Christopher's Hospice, Florence Wald shared issues involving the development of the Connecticut Hospice, and Dr Balfour Mount spoke of the development of the Palliative Care Unit of the Royal Victoria Hospital in Montreal (Vachon, 1999).

The 1970s: a time of change

The sexual revolution had begun in the 1960s; homosexuality and heterosexuality were more openly discussed than they had been in previous generations. AIDS was an unknown phenomenon. The values of society were being seriously questioned, especially by its younger members, who coined the slogan 'Don't trust anyone over 30.'

> There was arrogance about having conquered many of the diseases known to society. Arnold Toynbee was quoted as saying that death was 'Un-American' (Stoddard, 1978). Technology was supreme and death was going to be overcome. Those who died were isolated in rooms at the end of the corridor. It was commonly stated that sex had come out of the closet, now it was time for death to come out of the closet. It was time to talk about death, to acknowledge that people did die and to improve the care of the dying. (Vachon, 1999, p. 231)
>
> In the early 1970s the Vietnam War was drawing to a close. Some of the younger people in the early days of the hospice movement had been involved in dodging the draft, others had been conscientious objectors, or had been in the war and were forever touched by it. Many were challenging the traditional beliefs of society. With the Vietnam War and nearly universal access to television in the United States and Canada, for the first time death had come into homes as a nightly occurrence on the 6 o'clock news. There was a desire to make death more meaningful than death in Vietnam and death in highly technological hospitals seemed to be. (Vachon, 1999, p. 232).
>
> In addition, consumers had become more active in the 1960s and 1970s. The self-help movement was flourishing. The Women's Movement was in full swing. Nurses were expanding their roles and attempting to become more collaborative partners with physicians (Vachon, Lyall, and Rogers, 1976). Women were becoming more assertive and pushing to change the assumptions under which they had been living their lives. They were assuming an active role in childbirth and fighting to have partners present for deliveries. Births were sometimes taking place at home. As we were reclaiming a role in the natural process of birth, many also wanted to assume a more active role in the universal experience of death. As birth could occur at home or in more humane health care settings, so too might death occur at home, or in more home-like settings, such as hospices. (Vachon, 1999, p. 232)

Dr Robert Fulton, an early pioneer and leader in the field, often referred to the 'Female Trinity' of Dr Cicely Saunders, Dr Elisabeth Kübler-Ross, and Mother Theresa, the women who changed the face of the care of the dying as we knew it in the 1960s and 1970s.

Frameworks for studying occupational stress

From the early days in the field the most common outcome measures of occupational stress were, and still are, distress and burnout. Currently, commonly used terms are: stress, distress, or psychological morbidity (Ramirez, Graham, Richards, et al., 1995,

1996; Asai, Morita, Akechi, et al., 2007; Dougherty, Pierce, Ma, et al., 2009); burnout (Maslach, Schaufeli, and Leiter, 2001; Maslach, 2003; Alkema, Linton, and Davies, 2008), and compassion fatigue (Figley, 1995, 2002; Alkema et al., 2008; Sabo, 2008). Less commonly researched is the concept of moral distress (Austin, 2001; Weissman, 2009). The most commonly researched topics are distress and burnout, which will be the focus of this chapter.

Burnout

Burnout is a form of mental distress manifested in 'normal' people who have not suffered prior psychopathology, and who experience decreased work performance resulting from negative attitudes and behaviours (Maslach and Leiter, 2008).

Components of burnout

Burnout is a psychological syndrome in response to chronic interpersonal stressors on the job (Maslach, Schaufeli, and Leiter, 2001). The three key dimensions are:

Overwhelming **emotional exhaustion** (EE)—the basic *individual stress dimension* of burnout. It refers to feelings of being over-extended and depleted of one's emotional and physical resources. Exhaustion is the most widely and most thoroughly analysed and studied aspect of burnout. Exhaustion prompts action to distance oneself emotionally and cognitively from work, as a way to cope with work overload (Maslach and Leiter, 2008).

Feelings of **cynicism** and detachment from the job (**depersonalization**) (DP)—the *interpersonal context* dimension of burnout, refers to a negative, callous, or excessively detached response to various aspects of the job. It is an attempt to put distance between oneself and various aspects of the job. Research shows a consistent strong relationship between exhaustion and cynicism emerges from the presence of work overload and social conflict (Maslach and Leiter, 2008).

Sense of **ineffectiveness** and **lack of personal accomplishment** (PA)—the *self-evaluation dimension* of burnout refers to feelings of incompetence and a lack of achievement and productivity at work. PA arises more clearly from a lack of resources to get the work done (e.g., lack of critical information, lack of necessary tools, or insufficient time). It may be directly related to EE and DP, or be more independent (Maslach, 2003).

Compassion fatigue

The concept of compassion fatigue was developed by a nurse (Joinson, 1992) and then popularized by Figley (1995, 2002). It has attracted some attention in the field of palliative care (Garfield, Spring, and Ober, 1995; Keidel, 2002; Wright, 2004; Abendroth and Flannery, 2006; Sabo, 2008).

Compassion fatigue is described as being almost identical to post-traumatic stress disorder, except that it applies to those emotionally affected by the trauma of another (usually a client or family member) (Figley, 1995). Compassion fatigue is also known as secondary or vicarious traumatization (Figley, 1995, 2002). Compassion fatigue (Figley, 1995) has been used to describe a syndrome that shares some characteristics with burnout: depression, anxiety, hypochondria, combativeness, the sensation of being on 'fast forward', and an inability to concentrate.

Garfield, Spring, and Ober (1995) wrote about compassion fatigue in the context of AIDS/HIV and stated that, in contrast to one who has burned out, the caregiver with compassion fatigue can still care and be involved. Wright (2004), a clinical nurse specialist and trauma/bereavement counsellor working in an accident and emergency department in the United Kingdom, gives the following signs of compassion fatigue: 'no energy for it anymore,' 'emptied, nothing left to give,' 'not wanting to go there again,' 'feeling depleted in every dimension,' 'too many questions and no answers,' and 'why am I doing this?' One of the limitations of the concept of compassion fatigue is that it simply looks at the response of the individual to dealing with patients/clients and not factors from the work environment that may contribute to staff members experiencing manifestations of distress in one form or another. Suggestions for avoiding and dealing with compassion fatigue and burnout are given elsewhere in this book (see also Kearney, Weininger, Vachon, et al., 2009).

The early days of research on distress and burnout in hospice and palliative care

In 1974 our team, Dr Lyall, Joy Rogers, and I visited the Palliative Care Unit (PCU) of the RVH before the unit opened and at two- to three-month intervals over the first 15 months of the service's development. The stress of the PCU staff was compared with that of other staff at the hospital, as well as with the stress of the women in the studies of breast cancer and bereavement we were also researching.

Three months after the development of the palliative care unit, the nursing staff had scores on the Goldberg General Health Questionnaire (GHQ) (Goldberg, 1978) that were twice as high as those of the nurses on the other units and about half the score of women newly diagnosed with breast cancer. The scores of the palliative care staff were very similar to those of newly widowed women (9.4 vs. 10) (Lyall, Rogers, and Vachon, 1976; Lyall, Vachon, and Rogers, 1980). Over the following ten months the stress decreased to negligible levels. Analysis of the data showed that those who were most stressed left the PCU. Those who stayed had lower stress scores from the beginning. Stressors from interpersonal problems among staff and inadequate support from other staff declined over time. Other problems decreased but continued to be areas of concern: facing the death of a patient, difficulty dealing with families, and watching patients suffer. Some of the factors associated with staying or leaving the service included: being more religious, and being more 'venturesome' or 'spontaneous' as opposed to 'shy' on the 16 Personality Factor scale (Cattell, Eber, and Tatsuoka, 1970).

In the mid-1990s I reviewed all available studies of staff stress in hospice/palliative care (Vachon, 1995). In the largest study, which was conducted in the early days of the hospice movement and involved 1,281 staff surveyed for the National Hospice Study (Mor and Laliberte, 1984; Masterson-Allen, Mor, Laliberte, et al., 1985), the burnout rate was low, but was found to be more common in those under age 40, with a higher level of education, with long tenure, and who worked full time. The hospice staff had a mean score of 9.3 out of 36, compared with a score of 26.04 out of 63 for mental health workers (Masterson-Allen et al., 1985; Stout and Williams, 1983). These findings are fairly typical of many of the studies over the next three decades. However Ramirez et al. (1995) found burnout more common in those under 55, and Dougherty et al. (2009) found no difference in stress in those who worked full or part time.

An overview of stress and burnout in hospice/palliative care: from the beginning to the present

Reviews of the literature of stress in palliative care over the first quarter century of the field (Vachon, 1995) and from the early 1970s through the early 2000s (Vachon and Sherwood, 2007) found many studies which reported that staff working in palliative care had either less burnout and stress than other professionals or that they experienced no more stress than other healthcare professionals working with seriously ill and/or dying persons.

The fact that stress in palliative care may be less than in other specialties does not negate the stress that does occur. Earlier studies identified the use of drugs, alcohol, and suicidal ideation of hospice medical directors and matrons (Finlay, 1990). Hospice nurses were more anxious, with associated psychosomatic complaints, than hospital nurses, although the latter were more dissatisfied with their jobs (Cooper and Mitchell, 1990).

More recent studies confirm that palliative care specialists experience less stress and burnout than their oncology colleagues in the United Kingdom (Ramirez et al., 1995) and in Japan (Asai et al., 2007). In the UK study of cancer clinicians and palliative care specialists, the latter group generally reported the lowest mean percentage of items rated as contributing 'quite a bit' or 'a lot' to overall job stress. The estimated prevalence of psychiatric disorder in this study in the total group was 28 per cent, similar to that of a more recent study of 401 British specialist registrars in palliative medicine, medical oncology, and clinical oncology (Berman, Campbell, Makin, et al., 2007). Palliative care specialists were the least stressed (25 per cent) and clinical oncologists were the most stressed (32 per cent) in the Ramirez et al. (1995) study.

The percentage of the total sample of the UK cancer clinicians and palliative care specialists (Ramirez et al., 1995) reporting high levels of exhaustion on the Maslach Burnout Inventory was similar to that of the normative sample (31 vs. 33 per cent) (Maslach and Jackson, 1982). The highest percentage of emotional exhaustion was amongst clinical oncologists (38 per cent) and the lowest amongst palliative care specialists (23 per cent). Clinicians who felt insufficiently trained in communication and management skills had significantly higher levels of distress than those who felt sufficiently trained.

In the Japanese study (Asai et al., 2007) of clinical oncologists and palliative care physicians, 20 per cent had psychiatric morbidity, 22 per cent had a high level of emotional exhaustion, 11 per cent had a high level of depersonalization, and 62 per cent had a low level of personal accomplishment. Clinical oncologists showed significantly higher psychiatric morbidity than palliative care physicians (21 vs. 12 per cent; $p = 0.05$). In addition, clinical oncologists were more likely to have low feelings of personal accomplishment (65 vs. 53 per cent; $p = 0.05$). Confidence in having sufficient time to communicate with patients was significantly associated with all the burnout scales. Insufficient confidence in the psychological care of patients was associated with physician burnout rather than involvement in end-of-life care.

British palliative care nurses (Payne, 2001) experienced lower burnout than expected. Only 16 per cent of the UK palliative care nurses experienced emotional exhaustion compared with 37 per cent of the allied health personnel, including nurses in the study of staff working in Cancer Care Ontario clinics in Canada (Grunfeld, Whelan, Zitzelsberger, et al., 2000) and 29 per cent of the oncology nurses at Memorial Sloan Kettering Cancer Center (MSKCC) in New York (Kash, Holland, Breitbart, et al., 2000). Thirty-one percent of the British palliative care nurses (Payne, 2001) reported low personal accomplishment compared with 54 per cent of the Ontario allied health professionals (Grunfeld et al., 2000). Although the data from MSKCC (Kash et al., 2000) are presented with mean scores, rather than as a percentage of those who score high on the Maslach Burnout Inventory items, the nurses at MSKCC had significantly lower personal accomplishment scores than the oncologists and they scored below the mean for doctors and nurses in the United States (Maslach and Jackson, 1982).

It is possible that distress in palliative care may be increasing. Berman et al. (2007) studied UK registrars in medical oncology, palliative medicine, and clinical oncology and found that there was no significant difference in the percentage of 'caseness' across specialties, 26.3 per cent of the total sample experienced distress as measured by the 12-item GHQ, 11.3 per cent experienced depression on the SCL-D, and 4 per cent expressed suicidal ideation. There were, however, significant differences in the mean scores of the specialties, with medical oncologists having the highest mean scores on a number of measures of stressors.

A recent study comparing staff in oncology and palliative care at Princess Margaret Hospital, using an author-constructed questionnaire (Dougherty et al., 2009) found that 63 per cent reported experiencing 'a great deal' of stress at work. There was no difference in the distress reported by the oncology and palliative care staff.

A model for understanding occupational stress

Recent research on burnout has focused on the degree of match or mismatch between the person and six domains of the job environment. The greater the gap or mismatch between the person and the environment, the greater the likelihood of burnout. The greater the match or fit the greater the likelihood of engagement with work. Six areas of work life encompass the major organizational antecedents of burnout. These include workload, control, reward, community, fairness, and values (Maslach, Schaufeli, and Leiter, 2001).

Burnout arises from chronic mismatches between people and their work settings in some or all of these areas. The area of values may play a central mediating role for the other areas (Maslach, Schaufeli, and Leiter, 2001); although, for individuals at risk of burnout, fairness in the work environment may be the tipping point determining whether people develop job engagement or burnout (Maslach and Leiter, 2008).

Emotion–work variables (e.g., requirement to display or suppress emotions on the job, requirements to be emotionally empathic) account for additional variance in burnout scores over and above job stressors (Maslach, Schaufeli, and Leiter, 2001). The literature in palliative care will be reviewed using this model. (The following section is adapted from Vachon, 2006.)

Workload

Hospice staff initially prided themselves on having the time to spend with patients that was conducive to the best patient care. Current issues with managed care, the nursing shortage and fiscal restraint has changed this in many settings (Vachon and Huggard, 2010). Direct patient care activities have an impact on stress through a heavy workload of complex care, a shortage of staff, and an experienced lack of competence (van Staa, Visser, and van der Zouwe, 2000). Nurses working with critically ill and dying children in Hong Kong and Greece felt unable to provide quality care because of the shortage in nursing personnel. This added to their stress (Papadatou, Martinson, Chung, et al., 2001). However, Payne's study of UK palliative care nurses (2001) found that despite workload being a frequently reported stressor it was not related to burnout.

When palliative care specialists were compared with clinical and radiation oncologists, problems with 'feeling overloaded and its effects on home life' were found to be significantly greater for the medical and clinical oncologists than for the palliative care specialists. Depersonalization and high GHQ scores were also associated with being overloaded (Ramirez et al., 1995). Senior House Officers in United Kingdom hospices (Lloyd Williams, 2002) described their posts as stressful. In the most recent study of UK registrars (Berman et al., 2007), the occupational stressor with the highest mean score, and ranking as highest stressor for all three specialties, was 'being overstretched at times'. As in other studies the 'effect of hours of work on personal/family life' is an important stressor for specialists. Indeed the items with the highest scores appear to relate to the very issues in clinical practice one might expect these trainees to be concerned about, being competent in the face of conflicting demands on time.

In the study of palliative care and oncology staff at Princess Margaret Hospital (Dougherty et al., 2009), the top two variables predicting stress were greater perceived workload and insufficient time to grieve patients' deaths. A total of 52 per cent felt that their workload negatively affected patient care and more than 80 per cent felt that it affected the ability to provide emotional support for patients and compassionate end-of-life care. In all, 55 per cent stated they did not have sufficient time to grieve the death of a patient, and more than 30 per cent felt they did not have enough resources to cope with work-related stress. These findings did not differ between oncology and palliative care staff. Of interest is that previous research at the same oncology centre conducted over 30 years earlier was initiated because of staff grief and difficulty dealing with the emotional needs of patients and families. In that study nurses reported a lack of resource personnel and physicians reported 'a tremendous workload imposed by the prevalence of cancer, the increased life expectancy and chronic nature of the disease' (Vachon, Lyall, and Freeman, 1978, from Sabo and Vachon, in press). Over the years, the workload in palliative care seems to have increased, while the workload in oncology has been an issue for many years (Vachon, 1976; Vachon et al., 1978; Vachon, 1987).

Lack of control

The issue of control is related to inefficacy or reduced personal accomplishment. Mismatches often indicate that individuals have insufficient control over the resources necessary to do their work or insufficient authority to pursue the work in what they believe is the most effective manner (Maslach and Leiter, 1997). Caregivers consistently report having difficulty performing their jobs because of a lack of organizational resources (Vachon, 1976; Vachon et al., 1978; Vachon, 1987; Ramirez et al., 1995, 1996; Grunfeld et al., 2000; Dougherty et al., 2009).

Practices in some hospices led by fiscal constraints have raised increasing concern. Nurses are sometimes expected to perform procedures in the community without adequate supervision and training. When people are expected to assume responsibility with inadequate training, they have difficulty functioning (Coyle, 1997). While this finding was documented several years ago, one of my clients with advanced disease commented on a similar problem as I was preparing this chapter. The nurses assigned to do home visits had no idea how to deal with the patient's recently inserted chest tube.

Problems of control may also involve issues of personal safety. Nurses working in a hospice in South Africa were uncomfortable going into some settings, particularly at night. As a group they explored with administration the option of refusing to go into some areas. The hospice provided them with cell phones. Brainstorming together, the nurses suggested asking the police to accompany them if they were really uncomfortable visiting certain areas but felt they should visit for the sake of the patient (Vachon, 2001b).

Reward

In the early days of hospices physicians and nurses did their work as volunteers, which obviously could not continue indefinitely. The son of a pioneering hospice physician, Dr Bill Lamers, commented that at one point his father returned home from a patient with his payment, a car trunk full of pasta. His upset wife responded, 'we can't pay the bills with pasta'. When I approached Dr Lamers about using the story, he responded that while there were numerous financial problems, which also put strain on the marriage, 'nothing could replace the feelings of gratitude, the expressions of "thanks" I received from so many patients and their families'. None the less, there was no question that family members suffered as pioneers put in huge amounts of financially uncompensated time.

Lack of reward may be financial when one doesn't receive a salary or benefits commensurate with achievements, or lack of social rewards when one's hard work is ignored and not appreciated by others. The lack of intrinsic rewards (e.g. doing something of importance and doing it well) can also be a critical part of this mismatch. Issues with the financial reward for work were noted by physicians (Graham, Ramirez, Cull, et al., 1996; Asai et al., 2007). Low personal accomplishment and high stress was reported when there was a lack of resources to do one's work (Graham et al., 1996; Dougherty et al., 2009).

In the study by Ramirez and colleagues (1995), the researchers found that when oncologists derived little satisfaction from their work they were at greater risk for experiencing burnout. In Huggard's (2008) study of 464 New Zealand staff working in palliative care, a number of respondents spontaneously mentioned that it was not the financial reward of the work that kept them in the field.

Community

This mismatch arises when people lose a sense of personal connection with others in the workplace. Social support from people with whom one shares praise, comfort, happiness, and humour affirms membership in a group with a shared sense of values (Maslach, Schaufeli, and Leiter, 2001; Maslach, 2003; Vachon and Sherwood, 2007). From fairly early in the field of palliative care the team was seen simultaneously as being a major stressor, the place where stress was manifest, and the group to whom one turned for support (Vachon, 1987). Team communication problems have long been identified as an issue in palliative care, as in other specialties. These have occurred across time and cultures and have been documented elsewhere (Vachon, 1987, 1995; Vachon and Sherwood, 2007; Vachon and Huggard, 2010).

In the early days of the hospice movement it was not unusual for pioneers to find themselves removed from their positions in the hospices they founded. While pioneers are often not the people to continue to grow an organization, these experiences often left pioneers feeling quite traumatized.

Stephen Connor, formerly of the National Hospice and Palliative Care Association and now with the World Palliative Care Association, has commented on issues with some of the conflict in hospice/palliative care. He says that 'hospice workers have been often described as angels. The burden of being so present and pure for our patients and families facing death for some has a consequence. As Jung observed there can be a shadow side to human personality. In healthcare generally and in hospice care especially some express that shadow in relations with co-workers' (Connor, 2010).

Studying hospice nurses in the United Kingdom, Payne (2001) found that dealing with death and dying, inadequate preparation, and workload were slightly more problematic than were conflict with doctors, conflict with other nurses, lack of support, and uncertainty concerning treatment. However, in that study conflict with staff contributed to both the emotional exhaustion and depersonalization subscales of the Maslach Burnout Inventory. More recently palliative care specialist registrars in the UK were more likely than oncology registrars to report finding stress from low prestige of their specialty and from difficulties with nursing staff (Berman et al., 2007).

Although teamwork has been seen as being the best, and perhaps only, way of doing palliative care, some of the assumptions of palliative care teamwork have come into question (Speck, 2006). A group consists of 'two or more people who are interacting with one another, who share a set of common goals and norms which direct their activities, and who develop a set of roles and a network of affective relationships' (Speck, 2006, p. 8). In contrast, a team is a group of people brought together, from within or outside of the organization, for a specific purpose or task. In working to achieve the task, it is expected that team members will work interdependently and take some ownership for the task. The quintessential feature of a small, well-balanced team is leadership that is shared or rotates, depending on the issue involved. Palliative care teams generally function with an identified leader, and there are often prescribed ways of dealing with issues such as standing orders. (Speck, 2006, in Vachon and Mueller, 2009). One team which is attempting to change some of the usual team approaches to providing care is the San Diego Hospice in California (2007). There, nurses, social workers, and chaplains all meet the patient/family when they come onto the service and together establish relationships and plan and provide care. An example they used to describe their care provision (von Gunten, personal communication, 2007) was that a chaplain would go to a patient's home. The patient might say that he was not particularly interested in speaking with a chaplain, what he really needed was a urinal. The chaplain would have a urinal in his car trunk, which he could provide. After some basic needs were met, the patient might or might not be interested in availing himself of the chaplain's more traditional services.

Research on a new palliative care team in an academic palliative care unit in Germany (Jünger, Pestinger, Elsner, et al., 2007) found that factors crucial to communication in the team members' views were close communication, team philosophy, good interpersonal relationships, high team commitment, autonomy, and the ability to deal with death and dying. Close communication was by far the most frequently mentioned criterion for cooperation. Team performance, good coordination of workflow, and mutual trust underpin the evaluation of efficient teamwork. Inefficient teamwork is associated with the absence of clear goals, tasks, and role delegation, as well as a lack of team commitment. The team members spoke of common understandings; mutual openness, respect, and a positive attitude; a basic trust in one another's contribution to the common goal; reliance on colleagues; and openness and flexibility. A lack of communication and task conflict were the most frequently mentioned factors requiring cooperation. However, at the end of the first year of operation, the three salient outcome criteria for cooperation— team commitment, work satisfaction, and team performance—had evolved positively in the view of the team.

Fairness

This mismatch arises when there is no perceived fairness in the workplace. Fairness communicates respect and confirms people's self-worth. Mutual respect between people is central to a shared sense of community. Recent research in a university setting showed that fairness in the work environment may be the tipping point determining whether people develop job engagement or burnout (Maslach and Leiter, 2008) A lack of fairness was perceived in unrealistic expectations of the organization(Vachon, 1987). There are concerns about funding rivalries between hospices and other settings of care (Webster and Kristjanson, 2002) and rivalries between different hospices have long been an issue (Vachon, 1987, 2006, from Sabo and Vachon, in press).

Barbara Monroe, a social worker with a long history of working in palliative care, and now CEO of St Christopher's Hospice, suggests there needs to be considerable change in the delivery of palliative care. She notes that a review of the literature suggests that the effectiveness of multi-professional teams in delivering palliative care has never really been addressed. She concludes that multi-disciplinary teams may have 'developed in part as a result both of shortcomings in the skill base of individual professionals, and a determination on the part of professionals to hold onto and reinforce the boundaries that determine and create their power' (Monroe and Speck, 2006, p. 203).

She observes that in moving forward, it will be important to assess the impact of recent initiatives such as nurse prescribing, nurse consultants and community matrons.

Monroe notes that in the National Health Service, quality and value for money are now dual goals, not alternatives. She warns that managing cost effectiveness will call into question the routine delivery of palliative care by multi-professional or interdisciplinary teams and she warns that we must be ready to meet this challenge. Also, in a resource-strapped future, there will be more attention paid to creating partnerships with outside agencies and an increased focus on cost-effectiveness (Monroe and Speck, 2006, from Vachon and Mueller, 2009). Part of this focus on cost effectiveness may come with a cost to staff members. While writing this chapter the author was consulted by a nurse with a dying family member who worked for a health-care agency. The nurse had great difficulty negotiating attending medical appointments with her dying family member, while continuing to do her job. She said the agency used to be flexible but with cost containment all they cared about was the 'bottom line'.

Monroe suggests there will be a move towards the standard palliative care package being delivered by 'well-resourced, multi-skilled, individual professionals, most often clinical nursing specialists, who have access to a team of experts for consultation' (Monroe and Speck, 2006, p. 206). With the changes being proposed (Monroe and Speck, 2006) it will be required to focus on 'first principles,' what it is that needs to be done for the highest and best good of the patients and the families whom we serve.

Values

People might feel constrained by their job to do something unethical and not in accord with their own values. Alternatively, there may be a mismatch between their personal career goals and the values of the organization. People can also be caught in conflicting values of the organization, as when there is a discrepancy between a lofty mission statement and actual practice, or when the values are in conflict (e.g. high-quality service and cost containment do not always coexist). Staffing problems can lead to not being able to do the job properly, a decrease in quality patient care and decreased staff morale (Grunfeld et al., 2000).

Initially those attracted to hospice/palliative care felt they were able to do work which was congruent with their value system. There were challenges, however, when others would not refer in what they thought was a timely fashion (Vachon, 1987), and this has continued to be an issue to the present time. With the changes Monroe suggests it is not likely that the problem will disappear.

Dr David Weissman (2009) recently wrote about moral distress and said, 'Since the service began in 1993 we have had two nurses and two physicians, with an accumulated 30-plus years of palliative care experience, partly or completely hang up their palliative care shingle. Paraphrasing their words, "I just can't do it anymore, I am so angry with the system I can't meet the needs of patients in a manner that lets me sleep at night"' (p. 865). Weissman points out that many pioneers were drawn to the field because of the gulf between actual and ideal care of patients they experienced during their formative years of training and practice. Speaking from his own experience he notes this occurred in the 1980s, but as we saw earlier, the same situation was what drew the earlier pioneers from the 1970s to the field. He says that for many of the early pioneers,

> moral distress was their 'emotional baseline,' a state that has both positive and negative effects. The positive has been the continued motivation to work to improve the system of care; the negative being the emotional toll on ourselves and our families. I think it is very healthy that many of the younger generation of palliative care clinicians have entered the field out of the desire to expand the research base, work to provide cutting edge education, and develop robust clinical programs, all for their own sake, rather than out of moral distress. (Weissman, 2009, p. 866)

For oncologists, the optimization of career fit (balance between personal and professional goals/values) has led to increased job satisfaction (Vachon, 1987; Shanafelt, Chung, White, et al., 2006).

Emotion–work variables

Emotion–work variables require the individual to display or suppress emotions on the job and involves the requirement to be emotionally empathic. Research has found these emotional factors account for additional variance in burnout scores over and above job stressors (Maslach, Schaufeli, and Leiter, 2001). Although the literature has been somewhat divided as to whether or not the care of the dying is a major stressor in hospice palliative care (Vachon, 1987, 1995), Payne (2001) found that the most problematic stressor reported by hospice nurses was 'death and dying.' In contrast, a survey of 464 palliative care staff of a variety of disciplines in New Zealand (Huggard, 2008, in Vachon and Huggard, 2010) did not identify 'death and dying' issues as a major contributor to creating a stressful work environment. Participants reported that these issues were manageable as long as there were sufficient and appropriate organizational support practices, such as acknowledgement of the deaths, the use of rituals, and the availability of debriefing, if required.

Boston, Towers, and Barnard (2001) noted that dying persons experience disruption of the essence of day-to-day living and challenges to their perception of who they are. Through this process, they gain new wisdom and reshape their sense of meaning in life. A different way of knowing the world evolves, characterized by inner know-how and tacit knowledge that defines the self in relationship to others. Caregivers and others around them 'are perceived to be in another place, or don't seem to be there at all' (p. 248). Patients and caregivers may feel that they just don't connect. Boston and co-authors (2001) speak of palliative care as taking caregivers into emotional realms that are neither easy nor comfortable. When patients experience meaning and peacefulness in relation to their approaching death, this enriches the lives of the clinicians involved. This phenomenon appears similar to the 'healing connections' identified by Mount, Boston, and Cohen (2007) in a study of terminally ill persons contrasting persons experiencing suffering and anguish during the dying process with those experiencing integrity and wholeness. This connection involves connection to self, others, the phenomenal world, and ultimate meaning.

Barnard et al. (2000) note that 'Palliative care is whole-person care not only in the sense that the whole person of the patient (body, mind, spirit) is the object of care, but also in that the whole person of the caregiver is involved. Palliative care is, par excellence, care that is given through the medium of a human relationship' (p. 5). Yet caregivers are not always able to engage in such relationships. Ramsay (2006), a psychiatrist and ceramic artist, did an observation study on a palliative care unit reported by Speck (2006). She noted that the presence of an observer went against a culture where emotions were shuttered off. The unit's philosophy, while not religious, was supported by butterfly badges and emblems. The tendency to shut off emotions was most marked in the way in which the body was removed from the ward, the lack of use of the communal day room, and the emphasis on privacy in people's rooms. Ramsay observes that both staff and patients in such a unit are faced with the dilemma of maintaining 'warm human contact that truly expresses the reality of facing death, while at the same time keeping sufficient distance to prevent being overwhelmed by it' (Ramsay, 2006, p. 93).

Georges, Grypdonck, and De Casterle (2002) studied nurses on an academic palliative care unit in Holland which was having trouble retaining nurses. They found two methods of practice described the nurses' actual activity. The first and more prominent method was 'striving to adopt a well-organized and purposeful approach as a nurse on an academic ward' ($n = 12$); the second was 'striving to increase the well-being of the patient' ($n = 2$). Nurses in the first group tended to take a 'scientific' perspective towards nursing diagnosis and their interactions with patients. They felt that the gravity of caring for dying patients would inevitably lead to burnout, so they did not plan to work too long in palliative care. They tended to distance themselves from patients by focusing on tasks and the treatment of symptoms. Some explained that their experience had taught them to remain more professional and detached while others decided consciously not to invest too much in their relationship with patients because it would be too demanding.

Dr Harvey Chochinov has developed 'dignity therapy' for use with the dying. In a forthcoming book (Chochinov, in press) he speaks of the importance of 'care tenor', the tone of care that healthcare providers offer patients or the tone that patients perceive. Care tenor denotes everything we convey to patients, beyond mere words. Care tenor should connote *You matter*. He suggests caregivers should think of themselves as being akin to a mirror. 'With every clinical contact, patients gaze our way, looking for an affirming reflection in which they can recognize themselves. If all they see is their illness, they may feel that the essence of who they are has vanished' (Chochinov, pre-publication, p. 30). While palliative care providers might think of themselves as always giving the message *You matter*, the distancing from patients and focusing on tasks in the Georges et al. (2002) study may inadvertently give the message to patients that they do not matter.

Coping: what keeps us going in our work?

Personal coping strategies

Being able to truly care for patients requires being able to care for ourselves. Internal medicine residents with increased mental well-being had increased empathy towards patients and practised more personal wellness promotion strategies (aspects of self-care, relationships, work attitudes, religious/spiritual practice, personal philosophies, and strategies related to work–life balance). (Shanafelt, West, Zhan, et al., 2005). In a study of close to 600 caregivers around the world (Vachon, 1987) the primary coping mechanisms that allowed caregivers to continue working with the critically ill, dying, and bereaved were: a sense of competence, control and pleasure in one's work; team philosophy, building, and support; control over aspects of practice; lifestyle management; and a personal philosophy of illness, death, and one's role in life. A more recent study of medical oncologists (Shanafelt, Novotny, Johnson, et al., 2005) had very similar findings. Half of the oncologists studied reported high overall well-being. Those with overall high well-being were more likely to be aged 50 or younger, male, working 60 hours or less per week, and engaging in personal wellness promotion strategies including: developing an approach/philosophy to dealing with death and end-of-life care, using recreation/hobbies/exercise, taking a positive outlook, and incorporating a philosophy of balance between personal and professional life. Oncologists with high overall well-being also reported greater career satisfaction.

A more recent study by Shanafelt's group of palliative care physicians (Swetz, Harrington, Matsuyama, Shanafelt, et al., 2009) surveyed 40 palliative care physicians, 30 of whom responded in full. Each listed from 1 to 7 strategies with a median of 4 per respondent. Physical well-being was the most common strategy reported (60 per cent), followed by professional relationships (57 per cent), taking a transcendental perspective (43 per cent), talking with others (43 per cent), hobbies (40 per cent), clinical variety (37 per cent), personal relationships (37 per cent), and personal boundaries (37 per cent). 'Time away' from work (27 per cent), passion for one's work (20 per cent), realistic expectations and use of humour and laughter (13 per cent each), and remembering patients (10 per cent) were cited less frequently (p. 773).

We enjoy our work and are good at it

There has been increasing attention to what brings caregivers satisfaction in their work as opposed to simply looking at problems and stressors. The benefits attributed to working with advanced cancer patients or individuals at the end of life include compassion satisfaction, job engagement, and satisfaction and counter-transference.

Compassion satisfaction is defined as 'the pleasure you derive from being able to do your work well' (Stamm, 2009, p. 12). Compassion satisfaction is the opposite of compassion fatigue. Job engagement is conceptualized as being the opposite of burnout (Maslach, 2003). It involves energy, involvement, and efficacy. Engagement involves the individual's relationship with work. This includes a sustainable workload, feelings of choice and control, appropriate recognition and reward, a supportive work community, fairness and justice, and meaningful and valued work. Engagement is also characterized by high levels of activation and pleasure (Maslach, 2003; Stenmarker, Palmerus, and Marky, 2009). Engagement is defined as a persistent, positive-affective-motivational state of fulfilment in employees that is characterized by vigour, dedication, and absorption (Maslach, 2003).

Relationships continue to remain at the core of supportive and palliative care. Katz (2006) has applied the psychiatric concept of counter-transference to end-of-life care. Counter-transference is defined as 'an "abbreviation" for the totality of our responses to our work—emotional, cognitive and behavioral—whether prompted by our patients, by the dynamics incumbent to our helping relationships, or by our own inevitable life experiences' (Katz, 2006, p. 6). End-of-life care professionals of all disciplines and levels of experience, not just therapists, are subject to powerful reactions to their work. These reactions are seen as being far more diverse than 'compassion fatigue' or 'vicarious traumatization'. Drawing on the quantum physics concepts which suggest that the whole is greater than the sum of its parts, similar to Kearney's *A Place of Healing: Working with Suffering in Living and Dying* (Kearney, 2000), Katz (2006) speaks of the alchemical reaction which occurs when two individuals engage together at the most vulnerable time in human existence—the end of life. Alchemy is 'that space' that takes its own place in the poignant relationship between helper and patient. Through the experience, both can be transformed (from Vachon and Mueller, 2009; Sabo and Vachon, in press).

Vitality has been defined as 'the capacity to live and develop or the power to endure' (*Merriam Webster Dictionary*, 2004). The concept has considerable relevance when considered within the context of supportive oncology and palliative care. Physicians, nurses, and other professionals have identified a 'way of living' through personal connections, significant emotional experiences, and meaning as underlying vitality (Webster and Kristjanson, 2002). Further, vitality has been associated with energy, life, animation, and importance. These very qualities may help to explain why many healthcare professionals reap immense rewards and personal satisfaction from their work, even in the face of patient/family suffering, trauma, and death (Sabo and Vachon, in press).

Webster and Kristjanson (2002) found that the lessons healthcare professionals learned from their work added meaning to their personal and professional lives. Described in terms of personal growth, the interactions with patients, families, and colleagues added a dimension to palliative care work that shifted their work beyond mere care (the technical aspect) to caring. Crucial to the experience of palliative care for the participants were patient and family, holistic care, and the interdisciplinary team (Webster and Kristjanson, 2002; from Sabo and Vachon, in press).

Personality constructs

The personality constructs of *hardiness* (commitment, control, and challenge) (Kobasa, 1979; Kobasa, Maddi, and Kahn, 1982); a *sense of coherence*, which sees one's life as being comprehensible, manageable, and meaningful (Antonovsky, 1987); and *resilience*, the ability to bounce back or cope successfully despite considerable adversity (Walsh, 2006), have been studied and found to be helpful in palliative and supportive care (Kash et al., 2000; Ablett and Jones, 2007; Monroe and Oliviere, 2007). Comparing the concepts of hardiness and a sense of coherence, which are associated with resilience, Ablett and Jones (2007) note that Hardiness is associated with resilience for some palliative care nurses, while a sense of coherence is associated with resilience for others. The key difference is response to change. Those who exhibit hardiness welcome change and those with a sense of coherence do not. This article is one of a few recent publications which recognizes that programmes of intervention are going to need to be different for different staff members. Redinbaugh, Schuerger, Weiss, et al. (2001)

note that there must be awareness that different team members may have different ways of dealing with emotionally challenging situations such as grief. Physicians and nurses may prefer different coping strategies and may have different personality structures that lead to different responses to patient deaths. Individuals have natural propensities and aversions for minimizing grief reactions. Some caregivers are likely to talk with others about their grief. Others attempt to understand their grief through its depiction in literature and the arts. Some might dampen their grief with alcohol or drugs, while others use personal faith to resolve their grief.

The power of positive emotion

Vaillant (2008) writes of the transformative power of positive emotion—compassion, forgiveness, love, hope, joy, faith/trust, awe, and gratitude. He notes that these arise from our inborn mammalian capacity for unselfish parental love. 'All human beings are hardwired for positive emotions, and these positive emotions are a common denominator of all major faiths and of all human beings' (Vaillant, 2008, p. 3). He suggests that such positive emotions are essential to the survival of *Homo sapiens* as a species. In contrast, negative emotions such as anger and fear are 'all about me' and do little to support growth and change within the individual, in part because of the focus on the present. Vaillant (2008) suggests that positive emotions are more expansive and help us to build. 'They widen our tolerance, expand our moral compass, and enhance our creativity. They help us to survive in time future . . . while negative emotions narrow attention and miss the forest for the trees. Positive emotions, especially joy, make thought patterns more flexible, creative, integrative and efficient' (p. 5).

Positive emotions have the capacity to undo the physical effects associated with negative emotions returning the individual to a pre-stressor baseline (Fredrickson, Mancuso, Branigan, et al., 2000). Positive emotions 'serve not only as breathers, providing a psychological break or respite, but also as restorers, replenishing resources' (Fredrickson, Tugade, Waugh, et al., 2003, p. 366). Research has found positive emotions to be associated with resilience, defined as the ability to bounce back or cope successfully despite considerable adversity (Walsh, 2006). Reinforcing the connection between positive emotions and resilience are the positive attributes of resilience such as 're-integration', sense of purpose or self-determination, positive relationships/a social network, flexibility, and self-esteem/self-efficacy (Earvolino-Ramirez, 2007). Resilient people may use positive emotions as a mechanism for coping (from Sabo and Vachon, in press).

Baumrucker, a palliative care physician, wrote of his experience of transformation in palliative care (2002). He was proud of the fact that he hadn't taken any vacation time in seven years and took out large insurance policies so his colleagues could benefit if he was killed on a professional trip, not caring whether he lived or died.

> I took a grim satisfaction out of fulfilling all of the requirements expected of me, and I bragged that I didn't need time off or any other 'silly things like that.' What I didn't realize for years was that I was also practicing medicine like a machine. Although I looked human on the outside, I was practicing a soulless medicine, all science and very little heart. I was irritable in my medical practice but did manage to find some respite in hospice care. (Baumrucker, 2002, p. 155)

Things changed when he met a woman, married, and began to enjoy life. 'I was turning down work because I cared about my free time. I realized I couldn't give compassionate care to my patients until I was compassionate with myself' (p. 155). He became suddenly aware of his shift when he heard a colleague speak about stress in hospice and the way in which peak athletes are trained in a manner which involves the whole person, including mental acuity, emotional health, physical conditioning, and spiritual well-being. The need for oscillation between energy expenditure (stress) and energy renewal (recovery) to maintain peak performance and improve quality of life was identified. Baumrucker (2002) can now 'generalize that a healthy psyche is necessary for peak performance in the workplace and at home' (p.155).

While caregivers may derive great satisfaction from their work, unless they refuel their own systems they will not be able to continue in the field (Kearney et al., 2009).

Conclusion

This chapter has been a selected review of literature from before the beginning of hospice/palliative care through to the present time. In the previously mentioned international study conducted in the early 1980s, before the days of AIDS/HIV (Vachon, 1987), when close to 600 caregivers to the critically ill, dying, and bereaved were interviewed, 100 of those interviewed were in hospice/palliative care. Of the stressors they reported, almost half (48 per cent) derived from the work environment; 29 per cent came from the occupational role, 17 per cent from patients and families, and 7 per cent from illness-related variables. The top stressors in palliative care were communication problems with others in the system; role ambiguity; team communication problems; communication problems with administration; role conflict; the nature of the system; inadequate resources; unrealistic expectations of the organization; patient/family communication problems and patient/family coping or communication problems.

Baumrucker (2002) speaks of burnout and says, '[g]iven the stresses in dealing with death-and-dying issues, paperwork, regulatory upkeep, distressed families, late or inappropriate referrals, and marginal reimbursement, it is no surprise that nurses, social workers, aides, chaplains, physicians, and all other hospice and palliative caregivers are at risk' (p. 154). These stressors and the ones noted above, particularly in the area of work overload, team communication issues, fairness, rewards, and the fact that the stressors in the recent study at Princess Margaret Hospital are similar to the stressors identified when I was first involved in studying stress in that institution with my colleagues, makes me wonder how much things have changed with regard to stress since the early days.

Weissman (2009) notes that many of the professionals involved in palliative care in the early days entered the field because of a moral distress about the way dying people were being treated and care was being provided. There is no doubt that in some ways care has improved, but in other ways care needs to continue to be improved. The fact that palliative care programmes initially did recognize that the work was potentially stressful and developed support groups and attention to staff needs may have led to staff stress being lower that that experienced by caregivers in other specialties, yet some of the current research (Berman et al., 2007) suggests that the stress of palliative care physicians, at least, may be increasing and that they are concerned about the status of their chosen field. It is not a time to be complacent.

As I finish this chapter I am attending a Dignity Therapy course with Dr Harvey Chochinov. The meeting has attracted people who have been in the field for many years, as well as some neophytes. The group is interdisciplinary and international and there is an excitement about bringing Chochinov's carefully researched concepts into clinical practice. Ample time is provided for spending time with one another, reflection, and self-care. Many people are excited about bringing new concepts back to their hospices and palliative care units, see themselves as being in units where new ideas are welcome, and seem to be experiencing the satisfaction and stimulation that will allow them to continue in the field for years to come. If we can continue to find new approaches to delivering quality care, with colleagues who are prepared to communicate and grow, and if we develop self-care and self-awareness strategies, we should be able to grow and thrive in our chosen field for years to come.

References

Abendroth, M and Flannery, J. (2006). Predicting the risk of compassion fatigue: A study of hospice nurses. *Journal of Hospice and Palliative Nursing*, **8**, 346–56.

Ablett, J. and Jones, R. (2007). Resilience and well-being in palliative care staff: a qualitative study of hospice nurses' experiences of work. *Psycho-Oncology*, **16**, 733–40.

Alkema, K., Linton, J., and Davies, R. (2008). A study of the relationship between self-care, compassion satisfaction, compassion fatigue, and burnout among hospice workers. *Journal of Social Work in End-of-Life and Palliative Care*, **4**, 101–19.

Antonovsky, A. (1987). *Unraveling the Mystery of Health: How People Manage Stress and Stay Well*. London: Jossey-Bass.

Artiss, K.L. and Levine, A. (1973). Doctor–patient relationships in severe illness. *New England Journal of Medicine*, **288**, 1210–14.

Asai, M., Morita, T., Akechi, T., et al. (2007). Burnout and psychiatric morbidity among physicians engaged in end-of-life care for cancer patients: A cross-sectional nationwide survey in Japan. *Psycho-Oncology*, **16**, 421–8.

Austin W. (2001). Nursing ethics in an era of globalization. *Advances in Nursing Science*, **24**, 1–18.

Barnard, D., Towers, A., Boston, P., and Lambrinidou, Y. (2000). *Crossing Over: Narratives of Palliative Care*. New York: Oxford University Press.

Baumrucker, S.J. (2002). Palliative care, burnout, and the pursuit of happiness. *American Journal of Hospice and Palliative Care*, **19**, 154–6.

Berman, R., Campbell, M., Makin, W., and Todd, C. (2007). Occupational stress in palliative medicine, medical oncology and clinical oncology specialist registrars. *Clinical Medicine*, **7**, 235–42.

Boston, P., Towers, A., and Barnard, A. (2001). Embracing vulnerability: Risk and empathy in palliative care. *Journal of Palliative Care*, **17**, 248–53.

Caplan, Gerald (1964). *Principles of Preventive Psychiatry*. New York: Basic Books.

Cattell, R.B., Eber, H.W., and Tatsuoka, M.M. (1970). *Handbook for the Sixteen Personality Factor Questionnaire (16 P F)*. Champaign, IL: Institute for Personality and Ability Testing.

Chochinov, H.M. (in press). *Dignity Therapy: Final Words for Final Days: A Handbook for Clinicians*. New York: Oxford University Press.

Cooper, C.L. and Mitchell, S. (1990). Nursing the critically ill and dying. *Human Relations*, **43**, 297–311.

Coyle, N. (1997). Focus on the nurse: Ethical dilemmas with highly symptomatic patients dying at home. *Hospice Journal*, **12**, 33–41.

Dougherty, E., Pierce, B., Ma, C., Panzarella, T., Rodin, G., and Zimmermann, C. (2009). Factors associated with work stress and professional satisfaction in oncology staff. *American Journal of Hospice and Palliative Medicine*, **26**, 105–11.

Earvolino-Ramirez, M. (2007). Resilience: A concept analysis. *Nursing Forum*, **42**, 73–82.

Feifel, H. (1950). *The Meaning of Death*. New York: Blakiston Division, McGraw-Hill.

Figley, C.R. (ed.) (1995). *Compassion Fatigue: Coping with Secondary Traumatic Stress Disorder in Those Who Treat the Traumatized*. New York: Brunner/Mazel.

Figley, C.R. (ed.) (2002). *Treating Compassion Fatigue*. New York: Brunner-Routledge.

Finlay, I.G. (1990). Sources of stress in hospice medical directors and matrons. *Palliative Medicine*, **4**, 5–9.

Folta, J. R. (1965). The perception of death. *Nursing Research*, **14**, 233–35.

Fox, R.C. (1959). *Experiment Perilous*. Glencoe, IL: The Free Press.

Fredrickson, B., Mancuso, R., Branigan, C., and Tugade, M. (2000). The undoing effect of positive emotions. *Motivation and Emotion*, **24**, 237–58.

Fredrickson, B., Tugade, M., Waugh, C., and Larkin G. (2003). What good are positive emotions in crises? A prospective study of resilience and emotions following the terrorist attacks on the United States on September 11th, 2001. *Journal of Personality and Social Psychology*, **84**, 365–76.

Fulton, R. (1965). *Death and Identity*. New York: John Wiley and Sons.

Garfield, C., Spring, C., and Ober D. (1995). *Sometimes My Heart Goes Numb: Love and Caring in a Time of AIDS*. San Francisco: Jossey-Bass.

Georges, J.J., Grypdonck, M., and De Casterle, B.D. (2002). Being a palliative care nurse in an academic hospital: A qualitative study about nurses' perceptions of palliative care nursing. *Journal of Clinical Nursing*, **11**, 785–93.

Glaser, B.G. and Strauss, A.L. (1964). Awareness contexts and social interaction. *American Sociological Review*, **29**, 669–79.

Glaser, B.G. and Strauss, A.L. (1965). *Awareness of Dying*. Chicago: Aldine.

Glaser, B.G. and Strauss, A.L. (1968). *Time for Dying*. Chicago: Aldine.

Goldberg, D. (1978). *Manual of the General Health Questionnaire*. Windsor: NFER-Nelson.

Graham, J., Ramirez, A., Cull, A., Finlay, I., Hoy, A., and Richards, M. (1996). Job stress and satisfaction among palliative physicians. *Palliative Medicine*, **10**, 185–94.

Grunfeld, E., Whelan, T.J., Zitzelsberger, L., Willan, A.R., Montesanto, B., and Evans, W.K. (2000). Cancer care workers in Ontario: prevalence of burnout, job stress and job satisfaction. *Journal of the Canadian Medical Association*, **163**, 166–9.

Health and Welfare Canada (1981). *Report of the Working Group on Special Services in Hospitals*. Ottawa: Health Services Directorate Health Services and Promotion Branch.

Hinton, J. (1967). *Dying*. Baltimore: Penguin.

Huggard, J. (2008). A national survey of the support needs of interprofessional hospice staff in Aotearoa/New Zealand. Master's thesis, University of Auckland, New Zealand.

Joinson, C. (1992). Coping with compassion fatigue. *Nursing*, **22**(4), 116–22.

Jünger, S., Pestinger, M., Elsner, F., Krumm, N., and Radbruch, L. (2007). Criteria for successful multiprofessional cooperation in palliative care teams. *Palliative Medicine*, **21**, 347–54.

Kash, K.M., Holland, J.C., Breitbart, W., et al. (2000). Stress and burnout in oncology. *Oncology*, **14**, 1621–37.

Katz, R. (2006). When out personal selves influence our professional work: An introduction to emotions and countertransference in end-of-life care. In R. Katz and T. Johnson (eds), *When Professionals Weep: Emotional and Countertransference Responses in End-of-life Care*. New York: Routledge, 3–12.

Kearney, M. (2000). *A Place of Healing: Working with Suffering in Living and Dying*. Oxford: Oxford University Press.

Kearney, M.K., Weininger, R.B., Vachon, M.L.S., Mount, B.M., and Harrison, R.L. (2009). Self-care of physicians caring for patients at the end of life: 'Being connected . . . a key to my survival'. *Journal of the American Medical Association*, **301**, 1155–64.

Keidel, G.C. (2002). Burnout and compassion fatigue among hospice caregivers. *American Journal of Hospital Palliative Care*, **19**, 200–5.

Klagsbrun, S. (1970). Cancer, emotions and nurses. *American Journal of Psychiatry*, **126**, 1237–44.

Kobasa, S.C. (1979). Stressful life events, personality and health: An inquiry into hardiness. *Journal of Personality and Social Psychology*, **37**, 1–11.

Kobasa, S.C., Maddi, S.R., and Kahn, S. (1982). Hardiness and health: A prospective inquiry. *Journal of Personality and Social Psychology*, **42**, 168–77.

Kübler-Ross, E.G. (1969). *On Death and Dying*. Toronto: Collier-Macmillan.

Lindemann, E. (1944). Symptomatology and management of acute grief. *American Journal of Psychiatry*, **101**, 141–8.

Lloyd Williams, M. (2002). Senior house officers' experience of a six month post in a hospice. *Medical Education*, **36**, 45–8.

Lyall, W.A.L., Rogers, J., and Vachon, M.L.S. (1976). Report to Palliative Care Unit of Royal Victoria Hospital regarding professional stress in the care of the dying. *Palliative Care Service Report*, Royal Victoria Hospital, Montreal, Quebec.

Lyall, W.A.L., Vachon, M.L.S., and Rogers, J. (1980). A study of the degree of stress experienced by professionals caring for dying patients. In I. Ajemian and B. Mount (eds), *The Royal Victoria Hospital Manual on Palliative/Hospice Care: A Resource Book*. New York City: ARNO Press, 489–509.

Maslach, C. (2003). Job burnout: New directions in research and intervention. *Current Directions in Psychological Scence*, **12**, 189–92.

Maslach, C., and Jackson, S.E. (1982). Burnout in health professions: A social psychological analysis. In G.S. Sanders and J. Suls (eds), *Social Psychology of Health and Illness*. London: Erlbaum, 227–51.

Maslach, C. and Leiter, M. (1997). *The Truth About Burnout: How Organizations Cause Personal Stress and What To Do About It*. San Francisco: Jossey-Boss.

Maslach C. and Leiter, M.P. (2008). Early predictors of job burnout and engagement. *Journal of Applied Psychology*, **93**, 498–512.

Maslach, C., Schaufeli, W.B., and Leiter, M.P. (2001). Job burnout. *Annual Review of Psychology*, **52**, 397–422.

Masterson-Allen, S., Mor, V., Laliberte, L., and Monteiro, L. (1985). Staff burnout in a hospice setting. *Hospice Journal*, **1**, 1–15.

Monroe, B. and Oliviere, D. (2007). *Resilience in Palliative Care: Achievement in Diversity*. New York: Oxford University Press.

Mor, V. and Laliberte L. (1984). Burnout among hospice staff. *Health and Social Work*, **9**, 274–83.

Mount, B., Boston, P., and Cohen, S. (2007). Healing connections: On moving from suffering to a sense of well-being. *Journal of Pain and Symptom Management*, **33**, 372–8.

Monroe, B. and Speck, P. (2006). Team Effectiveness. In P. Speck (ed.), *Teamwork in Palliative Care: Fulfilling or Frustrating?* Oxford: Oxford University Press, 201–9.

Papadatou, D., Martinson, I.M., Chung, P., and Man, M.N. (2001). Caring for dying children: A comparative study of nurses' experiences in Greece and Hong Kong. *Cancer Nursing*, **24**, 402–12.

Payne, N. (2001). Occupational stressors and coping as determinants of burnout in female hospice nurses. *Journal of Advanced Nursing*, **33**, 396–405.

Quint, J.C. (1966). Awareness of death and the nurse's composure. *Nursing Research*, **15**, 49–55.

Quint, J.C. (1967). When patients die: Some nursing problems. *Canadian Nurse*, **63**(12), 33–6.

Ramirez, A.J., Graham, J., Richards, M.A., et al. (1995). Burnout and psychiatric disorder among cancer clinicians. *British Journal of Cancer*, **71**, 1263–9.

Ramirez, A., Graham, J., Richards, M., Cull, A., and Gregory, W. (1996). Mental health of hospital consultants: The effect of stress and satisfaction at work. *Lancet*, **16**, 724–32.

Ramsay, N. (2006). Sitting close to death. In P. Speck (ed.), *Teamwork in Palliative Care: Fulfilling or Frustrating?* Oxford: Oxford University Press, 83–94.

Redinbaugh, E.M., Schuerger, J. M., Weiss, L., Brufsky, A., and Arnold, R. (2001). Health care professionals' grief: A model based on occupational style and coping. *Psycho-Oncology*, **10**, 187–98.

Rochester, S.R., Vachon, M.L.S., and Lyall W.A.L. (1974). Immediacy in language: A channel to the care of the dying patient. *Journal of Community Psychology*, **2**, 75–6.

Sabo, B. (2008). Adverse psychological consequences: Compassion fatigue, burnout and vicarious traumatization: Are nurses who provide palliative and haematological cancer care vulnerable? *Indian Journal of Palliative Care*, **14**, 23–9.

Sabo B. (2009). *Nursing from the Heart: An Exploration of Caring Work Among Hematology/ Blood and Marrow Transplant Nurses in Three Canadian Tertiary Care Centres.* Halifax: Dalhousie University.

Sabo, B. and Vachon M.L.S. (in press). Care of professional caregivers. In M.P. Davis, C. Zimmermann, P. Feyer, and P. Ortner (eds), *Supportive Oncology*. Philadelphia: Elsevier.

San Diego Hospice (August 2007). Shared Care FAQS.

Saunders, C. (1959). *Care of the Dying*. London: Macmillan.

Shanafelt, T., Chung, H., White, H., and Lyckholm, L. (2006). Shaping your career to maximize personal satisfaction in the practice of oncology. *Journal of Clinical Oncology*, **24**, 4020–6.

Shanafelt, T.D., Novotny, P., Johnson, M.E., et al. (2005). The well-being and personal wellness promotion strategies of medical oncologists in the North Central Cancer Treatment Group. *Oncology*, **68**, 23–32.

Shanafelt, T., West, C., Zhan, X. (2005). Relationship between increased personal well-being and enhanced empathy among internal medicine residents. *Journal of General and Internal Medicine*, **20**, 559–64.

Speck, P. (2006). *Teamwork in Palliative Care: Fulfilling or Frustrating?* New York: Oxford University Press.

Stamm, B. (2009). *The Concise Manual for the Professional Quality of Life Scale: The ProQOL*. Pocatello, ID: ProQOL.org.

Stenmarker, M., Palmerus, K., and Marky, I. (2009). Life satisfaction of Swedish pediatric oncologists: The role of personality, work-related aspects and emotional distress. *Pediatric Blood Cancers*, **53**, 1308–14.

Stoddard, S. (1978). *The Hospice Movement*. Briarcliff Manor, NY: Stein and Day.

Stout, J. and Williams, J. (1983). Comparison of two measures of burnout. *Psychological Reports*, **53**, 283–9.

Sudnow, D. (1967). *Passing On: The Social Organization of Dying*. Englewood Cliffs, NJ: Prentice-Hall.

Swetz, K.M., Harrington, S.E, Matsuyama, R.K., Shanafelt, T. D., and Lyckholm, L.J. (2009). Strategies for avoiding burnout in hospice and palliative medicine: Peer advice for physicians on achieving longevity and fulfillment. *Journal of Palliative Medicine*, **12**, 773–7.

Vachon, M.L.S. (1976). Staff stress in the care of the terminally ill. *Quality Review Bulletin*, May, 13–17

Vachon, M.L.S. (1978). Motivation and stress experienced by staff working with the terminally ill. *Death Education*, **2**, 113–22.

Vachon, M.L.S. (1987). *Occupational Stress in the Care of the Critically Ill, the Dying and the Bereaved*. New York: Hemisphere.

Vachon, M.L.S. (1995). Staff stress in palliative/hospice care: A review. *Palliative Medicine*, **9**, 91–122.

Vachon, M.L.S. (1999). Reflections on the history of occupational stress in hospice/palliative care. *The Hospice Journal*, **14**, 229–46.

Vachon, M.L.S. (2001a). One woman's thanatological journey. *Illness, Crisis & Loss*, **9**, 129–51.

Vachon M.L.S. (2001b). The nurse's role: The world of palliative care nursing. In B. Ferrell and N. Coyle (eds), *The Oxford Textbook of Palliative Nursing*. New York: Oxford University Press, 647–62.

Vachon, M.L.S. (2006). Staff stress and burnout in palliative care. In E. Bruera, I.J. Higginson, C. Ripamonti, and C.F. von Gunten (eds), *Textbook of Palliative Medicine*. London: Hodder Arnold, 1002–10.

Vachon, M.L.S. and Huggard, J. (2010). The experience of the nurse in end-of-life care in the 21st century: Mentoring the next generation. In B.R. Ferrell and N. Coyle (eds), *Textbook of Palliative Nursing*, 3rd edn. Oxford: Oxford University Press, 1131–56.

Vachon, M.L.S. and Lyall, W.A.L. (1976). Applying psychiatric techniques to patients with cancer. *Hospital & Community Psychiatry*, **27**, 582-4.

Vachon, M.L.S., Lyall, W.A.L., and Freeman, S.J.J. (1978). Measurement and management of stress in health professionals working with advanced cancer patients. *Death Education*, **1**, 365–75.

Vachon, M.L.S., Lyall, W.A.L, and Rogers, J. (1976). The nurse in thanatology: What she can learn from the woman's liberation movement. In A. Earle, N.T. Argondizzo, and A.H. Kutscher (eds), *The Nurse as Caregiver to the Dying Patient and His Family*. New York: Columbia University Press, 175–94.

Vachon, M.L.S., Lyall, W.A.L., Rogers, J., Cochrane, J., and Freeman, S.J.J. (1981–2). The effectiveness of psychosocial support during post-surgical treatment of breast cancer. *International Journal of Psychiatry in Medicine*, **11**, 365–72.

Vachon, M.L.S., Lyall, W.A.L., Rogers, J., Freedman, K., and Freeman, S.J.J. (1980). A controlled study of self-help intervention for widows. *The American Journal of Psychiatry*, **137**, l380–4.

Vachon, M.L.S. and Mueller, M. (2009). Burnout and symptoms of stress. In W. Breitbart and H. Chochinov (eds), *Handbook of Psychiatry in Palliative Medicine*. New York: Oxford University Press, 559–625.

Vachon, M.L.S. and Sherwood, C. (2007). Staff stress and burnout. In A.M. Berger, J.L. Shuster, and J.H. Von Roenn (eds), *Principles and Practice of Palliative Care and Supportive Oncology*. Philadelphia: Lippincott, Williams & Wilkins, 667–83.

van Staa, A.L., Visser, A., and van der Zouwe. (2000). Caring for caregivers: Experiences and evaluation of interventions for a palliative care team. *Patient Education and Counseling*, **41**, 93–105.

Vaillant, G. (2008). *Spiritual Evolution*. New York: Broadway Books.

Walsh, F. (2006). *Strengthening Family Resilience*. New York: Guilford Press.

Webster, J. and Kristjanson, L. (2002). 'But isn't it depressing?' The vitality of palliative care. *Journal of Palliative Care*, **18**, 15–24.

Weissman, D. (2009). Moral distress in palliative care. *Journal of Palliative Medicine*, **12**, 865–6.

Wright, B. (2004). Compassion fatigue: How to avoid it. *Palliative Medicine*, **18**, 4–5.

Chapter 2

Workplace well-being: a psychosocial perspective

Neil Thompson

Introduction

Workplace well-being is a subject that is receiving increasing attention these days (Thompson and Bates, 2009). A key part of well-being at work is the need to keep pressures within manageable limits and thus avoid stress. This chapter explores the importance of understanding stress as part of our developing awareness of workplace well-being. In particular, it emphasizes the importance of developing a *psychosocial* understanding of what is involved in making the workplace a humane and effective place.

Stress is commonly conceived as primarily an individualistic phenomenon. While it can clearly have major implications for individuals so affected, stress also has organizational and sociological dimensions. This chapter argues the case for placing a much stronger emphasis on the organizational (especially strategic) and social aspects of stress and its role in contemporary workplaces. It is argued that a failure to broaden our perspective on stress can lead to a highly distorted picture that fails to do justice to the complexities involved. This, in turn, has significant implications for both our theoretical understanding of stress and for policy and practice interventions in attempting to prevent and/or remedy stress and its harmful consequences as part of a commitment to workplace well-being.

The challenge of stress

Stress is a recurring theme in the management and organizational studies literature. It has been described as a 'buzz word' of the twenty-first century (DPP, 2006) and is widely recognized as a major problem in modern workplaces. It has also been dismissed as one big misunderstanding (or set of misunderstandings—see Patmore, 2006), although the criticisms levelled by this author relate more to the way in which stress issues have tended to be oversimplified by many people than to a genuine understanding of stress. Her conclusion that stress as a problem is overrated is therefore not a legitimate one.

Bunting (2004) helps us to understand just how significant stress is as an organizational challenge when she explains that:

> One in five British workers now reports that they have been affected by stress, and half a million people a year report stress levels that are making them ill. Work-related stress,

> depression and anxiety account for 13.4 million working days lost per year, more than any other work-related illness in the UK. People cite their jobs as the main cause of stress in their lives, well ahead of other worries such as money, family and health; in the Samaritans' 2003 survey 'Stressed Out', 36 per cent cited work as one of their biggest stressors. (p. 179)

This is just one of many sources that attest to the significant and growing impact of stress on both individuals and their employing organizations. However, not all organizations are taking the problem seriously, with many not having a policy on stress and even fewer monitoring and evaluating the effectiveness of that policy.

What adds to the difficulty is that, where the problems are being addressed, this is often in a narrow, individualistic way that does not do justice to the broader organizational or social factors involved. Many voices are now to be heard arguing for a move away from individualistic perspectives on stress towards organizational ones (Cranwell-Ward and Abbey, 2005; Sutherland and Cooper, 2000). None the less, dominant approaches continue to operate within a predominantly individualistic or 'atomistic' discourse (Thompson, 2010). As we shall see below, even authors who profess commitment to a broader approach easily revert to an individualistic perspective at times. The shift from a narrow, individualistic focus to a more holistic approach that takes account of both individual and organizational factors (and the vitally important interactions between the two) is something that is yet to happen in any significant way.

However, even if or when this shift takes place, there is still a very real danger that the focus will still be too narrow for two reasons. First, there is tendency for discussions of organizational matters to focus on operational dimensions at the neglect of the strategic. Even Sutherland and Cooper (2000), whose book carries the title of *A Strategic Approach to Stress*, maintain a focus primarily on operational matters. Little or no attention is paid to how stress relates to the ability or otherwise of an organization to achieve its strategic objectives and, of equal importance, how the pursuit of strategic objectives may give rise to, or at least exacerbate, stress. Second, this is because a psychological focus remains dominant, with little or no attention paid to wider sociological factors. As we shall see, there are distinct dangers involved in a reliance on 'psychologism'—a form of reductionism in which complex multi-level phenomena are reduced to matters of individual psychology. While such an approach is potentially very unhelpful in regard to *any* psychosocial phenomenon, it is particularly perilous in relation to stress, in so far as an over-emphasis on the individual dimension can produce a vicious circle of guilt, self-blame, and stigma that can make the situation significantly worse—for the individual concerned, as well as for the organization and its stakeholders (Thompson et al., 1994).

Broadening out the discussion to take account of organizational factors is clearly a step in the right direction, but it is important that:

(i) *the focus within organizations is strategic as well as operational.* If we neglect the strategic dimension, we omit consideration of a set of factors that can be highly significant.

(ii) *sociological aspects are also included in the picture.* Stress is not simply a matter of individual psychology; it is in large part shaped by social factors, and so any adequate understanding of it cannot afford to neglect the sociological dimension.

This chapter therefore seeks to:

(i) go beyond atomism in order to show the range of complex issues that exist above and beyond the level of specific employees;

(ii) go beyond the level of operations management and take account of the crucial role of strategy;

(iii) go beyond a psychological level to incorporate a sociological dimension within our understanding and analysis of stress; and

(iv) sketch out the implications of this broader perspective for dealing with stress as part of a commitment to workplace well-being.

Beyond individualism

The main problem with an individual model of stress from a theoretical point of view is that it tells only one part of the story. In seeking an adequate understanding of stress it would be a serious neglect of intellectual duty to fail to account for the social and organizational elements that can be seen to be very relevant (although, unfortunately, much of the theoretical work on the subject does precisely this).

The main problem with an individual model of stress from a policy and practice point of view is that it can be seen to be counter-productive. An individualized approach can leave people who experience stress feeling guilty and blaming themselves for a situation in which at least part of it (and possibly all of it) will be due to broader social and organizational factors, rather than individual ones. This can lead to stigma (stress comes to be seen as a sign of a weak or inadequate individual), shame, and a reluctance to address or even acknowledge the issues. This, in turn, can make the situation worse, unnecessarily increasing levels of stress.

Furnham and Taylor (2004), in writing about problematic behaviours at work, make the important point that: 'We are all psychologists in the sense that we choose to explain events at the level of the individual; not the group, not society as a whole but the individual' (p. 2). If we are to develop an adequate understanding of stress (and thus an adequate basis for tackling it), we need to move beyond a reliance on psychology alone and develop a broader psychosocial perspective that draws on both psychological and sociological insights (including the sociology of organizations).

However, despite this, a strong individualist focus persists. For example, Cranwell-Ward and Abbey (2005) quote the UK Health and Safety Executive (HSE) definition of stress, a definition which is closely linked to the HSE's emphasis on *organizational* issues—for example, in relation to the management standards they have identified (www.hse.gov.uk/stress/standards). However, the authors then go on to quote what they refer to as their 'favoured' definition, which is purely individualistic. This is particularly disappointing in a book that carries the title of *Organizational Stress*.

Cranwell-Ward and Abbey (2005) devote considerable space in Part 5 of their book to the individual aspects of stress. Part 4 addresses the organizational context, but predominantly from an individual perspective and without taking account of the strategic aspects of the organizational dimension. This book is by no means exceptional in adopting this approach. The literature generally tells only part of the story, and thereby sustains a discourse of atomism and thus of pathology. While this approach remains pervasive, stress will continue to be a significant and costly problem for individuals (and their families), for organizations (and all their stakeholders), and for the fabric of society more broadly.

Even a well-established text such as Earnshaw and Cooper (1996) draws primarily on an individual focus. For example, on page 8, they refer to the Cooper–Cummings framework and its emphasis on individual and behavioural symptoms of stress. As we shall see below, the use of the term 'symptom' is quite significant. Even where the focus moves on to organizational sources of stress (p. 15 onwards), the emphasis is still primarily on individual aspects of the organizational context. Many texts discuss the importance of support but, again, this tends to be conceptualized in individual terms, rather than addressing support as a broader set of issues about social relations. This reflects the tendency for support to be seen as an organizational fillip to assist the worker in his or her individual responsibility to fend off stress. The idea that, given the organizational nature and origin of much stress, employing organizations have a significant stake in making sure that stress is not allowed to develop is an important one, but sadly not one that is widely adopted.

However, one step in the right direction can be found in Sutherland and Cooper (2000), where they are critical of the focus on the individual:

> The Institute of Employment Studies (IES) research and recommendations, drawing on eight studies, including Marks and Spencer, the Nationwide Building Society, Nestlé, the Post Office, and South West Water, found that, all too often attention is focused on the individual, rather than on the individual as an element within the work environment. It was found that unfocused stress management systems have only a limited impact. (p. 3)

None the less, even within that same text, on page 62 there is a reference to a tripartite model for stress management in which the following three organizational elements are identified:

- To identify, eliminate, or minimize stressful situations.
- To teach the individual to cope with stress.
- To help those individuals who have become victims of exposure to stress.

While this contains elements of an organizational approach, as we shall see below, it certainly does not go far enough in drawing out the organizational implications of stress and remains too closely rooted to matters concerned with the individual worker (see also Korcszynski, 2007, for a critique of individualism in relation to stress).

The major reason for seeking to move beyond the level of the individual is that individualization has long been recognized as closely linked with the tendency to pathologize—that is, to regard the source of problems as being a deficit within the individual (Thompson et al., 1994), rather than recognize stress as a complex, multi-level phenomenon. An example of this would be the use of medical terminology that supports an individualized, medical model of stress, rather than a broader, multi-dimensional one. Such terminology includes the use of terms like 'symptoms' and 'treatment'. Of course, we *treat* a pathology, whereas stress interventions are (or should be) concerned with *intervening* in a complex, psychological, organizational, and social system and set of structures.

In this regard, the comments of Butt (2004) are quite helpful when he makes the important point that there is no isolated individual; that people have to be understood in terms of their social context. To fail to develop this broader perspective amounts to an example of the reductionism I referred to earlier:

> What makes social life interesting and valuable is that the whole interaction cannot be simply assembled from the parts. It is the organising of the parts into a meaningful gestalt that characterises interactions in the human order.
>
> It is this formulation of the social order that Blumer (1969) and Shotter (1993) refer to as 'joint action'. The outcome of a social act cannot be traced back to the individual intentions of any of the participants. (p. 122)

The work of Bauman (2001), an eminent sociologist, is quite relevant to our concerns here, even though he does not address stress directly. He argues that society has now entered a phase in which issues that were previously regarded as collective concerns are now increasingly being conceptualized in individualistic terms as a result of the uncertainties in the world of work. He links this with the relative demise of trade unions and their influence in tackling workplace problems. The modern workplace is one characterized by uncertainty and insecurity arising from an increasing emphasis on employment flexibility, and this can be seen to have the effect of developing a focus on individual approaches to problems rather than collective ones:

> The present-day uncertainty is a powerful *individualizing* force. It divides instead of uniting, and since there is no telling who might wake up in what division, the idea of 'common interests' grows ever more nebulous and in the end becomes incomprehensible. Fears, anxieties and grievances are made in such a way as to be suffered alone. They do not add up, do not cumulate into 'common cause', have no 'natural address'. (p. 24)

The decline in the notion of a 'job for life', then, undermines collective responses to common problems. In support of this conception of the modern workplace (Bauman refers to 'liquefied modernity' rather than postmodernity) is some recent research from Developing Patient Partnerships (DPP, 2006) in which 'change in financial state' was seen to have risen from a position of seventh in the Holmes and Rahe 'league table' of stress factors in 1967 to third in the 2006 survey ('job security' is fifth on the list).

Bauman's work is an important contribution to our understanding of the dangers of adopting too narrow and individualistic an approach, one that can be seen to 'blame the victim' (Ryan, 1988). Bauman again makes apt comment when he argues that:

> If they fall ill, it is because they were not resolute and industrious enough in following the health regime. If they stay unemployed, it is because they failed to learn the skills of winning an interview or because they did not try hard enough to find a job or because they are, purely and simply, work-shy. If they are not sure about their career prospects and agonize about their future, it is because they are not good enough at winning friends and influencing people and have failed to learn as they should the arts of self-expression and impressing the others. This is, at any rate, what they are told–and what they have come to believe, so that they behave 'as if' this was, indeed, the truth of the matter. As Beck

> aptly and poignantly puts it, 'how one lives becomes a *biographical solution to systemic contradictions.*' Risks and contradictions go on being socially produced; it is just the duty and the necessity of coping with them which is being individualized. (p. 47)

In short, the dominant thinking about personal troubles would appear to be at a disappointingly low level of sophistication, owing more to a tabloid mentality than a well-informed and carefully considered intelligent approach.

The picture, then, is a mixed one. There are still very strong signs of an individual focus, even in the literature that purports to focus on organizational matters, and where there is an emphasis on the organization, it remains primarily if not exclusively at an operational level. It is to this latter point—the relative absence of a strategic focus—that we now turn.

The strategic focus

The development of the Health and Safety Executive Management Standards in the UK for preventing and responding to stress can be seen as a helpful move away from individualism to a more holistic focus that incorporates the organizational dimension. We now need to build on such developments by taking the analysis further. One key part of this is to develop an emphasis on the strategic dimension of organizational life.

Clearly, an organizational focus on stress is important, but the argument presented here is that such an organizational focus needs to be strategic. Operational matters are important, but these are often led by the strategic underpinnings of the organization. Close attention therefore needs to be paid to the link between stress and strategy. Sutherland and Cooper (2000) profess a strategic approach to stress, but in reality their focus is almost exclusively operational. For example, on page 59 they distinguish between adaptive and maladaptive ways of coping, again reinforcing a pathological model of stress, leaving behind any consideration of the overall organizational strategy, its culture, and so on. On page 125, they write of the importance of an organizational approach, but there is no mention here of the strategic aspect of organizational life.

Organizational strategy is defined as:

> the direction and scope of an organisation over the long term, which achieves advantage for the organisation through its configuration of resources within a changing environment and to fulfil stakeholder expectations. (Johnson and Scholes, 2002, p. 10)

What is particularly relevant about this definition is the reference to 'the configuration of resources'. If we conceive of staff as *human* resources, then this notion gains additional significance, as it means that how an organization deploys, develops, and communicates with its employees will stem from their overall strategic approach. How staff are treated—and thus whether they are adequately supported and valued on the one hand or overloaded and undermined on the other—is therefore in large part a strategic consideration and not just an operational one.

There are three aspects of the strategic dimension of stress that I feel it is important to emphasize:

1. The importance of control in relation to stress has long been recognized in the stress literature. As Clutterbuck (2003) comments: 'In general, the more control

people have over when and how they work, the more that they feel they have balance in their lives' (p. 74). But here the emphasis is predominantly on individual control. There has been little or no mention in the literature of organizational control through strategy development and implementation and thus through leadership. This is a significant gap in our understanding. It continues to reinforce an individualized model and neglects the highly significant role of an organization's strategy. Control can be seen to be just as important at a strategic level as it is at an individual level, and so the dominant approach in the literature presents only one side of the story.

2. There has also been a long-standing emphasis on stress management training and this is predominantly concerned with helping individuals recognize stressors and develop their coping strategies. While there is no doubt much to commend this sort of training in some ways when it is carried out effectively, on its own it can be counter-productive, as again it can reinforce a pathological model, in so far as it fails to take account of the wider organizational matters. With regard to the strategic dimension, there is a significant gap in terms of a lack of emphasis on leadership training. I would argue that leadership training can be just as important, if not more so, as stress management training, because effective leaders can play a key part in developing workplaces where there is no culture of overwork or of the guilt that can arise through such problems as 'presenteeism' (where a culture has developed in which employees feel under pressure to work unnecessarily long hours—see Clutterbuck, 2003, p. 26). An effective leader can help to develop and sustain a culture of dignity at work where people are valued and morale is high (Bolton, 2007). This can play a significant role in terms of preventing stress, and again balances out the picture, so that the focus does not remain almost exclusively on the individual. A focus on leadership training can therefore help to move us away from the problem mentioned earlier—that of 'blaming the victim': holding the individual responsible for a range of factors, many of which will be beyond his or her control.

3. It has long been recognized that it is important to focus on attitudes as far as stress is concerned. Again, this is something that has not escaped the majority of people who are concerned with the challenge of stress in the workplace. However, the term 'attitudes' implies once again an individual issue. We can also see that it can be applied in relation to the strategic concern with organisational culture, in so far as a culture is in part a set of shared attitudes. Given that a key aspect of strategic management is the development of helpful and productive workplace cultures, strategic concerns should therefore include shaping attitudes. In other words, where attitude change is needed in order to prevent or remedy stress, this can be seen to be as much a strategic management responsibility as it is a matter for individual employees.

A person experiencing stress may have arrived at this situation in part as a result of his or her own actions, inactions, assumptions, or attitudes. However, it would be naive not to recognize that organizations also play an important role in the development of stressful situations. The development of a fuller organizational perspective on stress is therefore clearly called for, and what is also apparent is that such an organizational perspective needs to incorporate the strategic dimension and not stop at a consideration of operational matters. Senior managers need to ask themselves whether their strategy and its implementation help to prevent stress (for example, by valuing staff) or is perhaps instrumental in creating or exacerbating it (for example, by regarding staff as dispensable cogs in a machine, rather than a genuine human resource worthy of investment).

A sociological focus

Individuals do not exist in a social vacuum. Human experience can, in some respects, be seen to owe as much to wider issues of social context (social processes, structures, institutions, and influences) as to matters of individual actions. What is needed, then, is a *psychosocial* perspective—that is, one which incorporates both psychological and sociological insights.

Butt's (2004) comments are once again very helpful when he writes of a person–society dualism:

> The self is inside and society is outside. The psychological individual is then elevated into a position of primacy. This individual, it is claimed, is concrete, real for all to see, while society is an abstraction. Psychology studies individuals, while sociology focuses on society. In my view, this way of dividing up the field is highly problematic. . . . Psychology has moulded itself after the high-prestige natural science. No one disputes that society is made up of individuals and that individuals exist in the context of society. But individualism claims that, in an important sense, individuals precede society. Social psychology, that aspect of psychological science that deals with the social world, generally sees individuals as atoms that come together to produce and determine sociological phenomena. It acknowledges the existence of conformity, groupthink and obedience to authority, but sees these as puzzles to be explained primarily at the level of the individual. (pp. 16–17)

Butt is right to be critical of this perspective that neglects the highly significant role of the social context as a very relevant aspect of the situation (rather than simply a secondary backdrop to the assumed primary concern with individual psychology). One important thing that sociology has taught us is that society has a logic of its own, in the sense that it is not simply an aggregate of the actions of individuals. This can be seen to apply in terms of:

(i) the 'sedimented' meanings that are part and parcel of cultural formations. Baldwin (2004) refers to 'cultural sedimentation, whereby old meanings accumulate in our practices without our being aware of them' (p. 326). For example, what we regard as *personal* viewpoints will often be a reflection of our cultural upbringing (and therefore just as much social as individual).

(ii) institutionalized relations based on social structures. Class, gender, race, and ethnicity—these and many others are examples of how social relations, over time, become established as social structures and thus as social divisions (ways of dividing society up into sections and subsections, and thereby serving as a basis of social inequality). Durkheim, one of the founders of the discipline of sociology, pointed out that each of us is born into a society that precedes us (Durkheim,

1912). That is, we do not start life with a clean slate—much will already have been decided for us by our 'social location'. For example, those born into positions of poverty and deprivation will face significant disadvantages in terms of access to power and life chances compared with those born into affluence and social privilege. Much will depend on how we, as individuals, react to these social circumstances, but the significant influence of the social context in shaping our lives cannot be denied.

That is, while individuals are clearly important, each one is part of a very significant social context. To do justice to the complexities of stress, we need to take account of both individual factors and the wider sociological ones.

There are some key sociological factors that have received scant attention in the stress literature, and there is little sign that they are about to become a major focus of concern. These factors include:

◆ *Power relations*: These are very relevant in terms of such strongly stress-related issues as bullying and harassment on the one hand, and expectations on the other. In terms of the latter, we have the power to define expectations (which, if unreasonable or unclear, can be a significant source of stress), and in relation to what is known as internalized oppression (Thompson, 2003)—that is, where people have internalized expectations of themselves that are unrealistic due to the pressures of the prevailing culture or of particular individuals.

◆ *Social divisions*: Such factors as class, race, and gender can be very significant in terms of: (i) what is perceived as a stressor; (ii) what coping methods are adopted; and (iii) how support is used. For example, black people are likely to face pressures brought about by racism and thus face challenges in terms of how they cope with such pressures, while the support available may vary considerably—perhaps depending on whether or not there are white colleagues who are prepared to work with black colleagues as part of an anti-racist alliance.

◆ *Culture*: There are distinct cultural differences in terms of how people respond to life in general, and so it would be highly surprising to find that culture is not relevant to stress issues, and, of course, there is also the dimension of organizational culture, as discussed earlier.

◆ *Discourse*: How language is used can be very significant in terms of how stress is conceptualized. For example, if it is presented as a matter of individual pathology, we should not be surprised to find that many people will not seek help and the problem may therefore escalate without appropriate interventions being carried out at the key time.

These are just an indicative range of a number of sociological factors that have a bearing on stress. The continued focus almost exclusively on psychological dimensions is clearly, therefore, quite counter-productive in developing an adequate theoretical model of stress, and therefore an adequate basis for tackling the problems that stress presents.

By incorporating a sociological dimension to our studies of stress, we can begin to broaden our outlook by, for example, developing our research focus from personal matters to include also organizational/strategic matters and, indeed, wider societal ones. This can involve a focus on qualitative research studies as well as the more common quantitative ones. Quantitative research is well suited to providing a picture of psychological matters but, if we are to have a fuller understanding of how the individual experiences the wider social world, we need the depth that qualitative analysis can bring to academic research.

Earlier studies of stress began with an engineering analogy (for example, the work of Selye, 1956), based on the idea of excessive pressure producing strain on a structure (a bridge, for example). From this there developed an 'appraisal' model (in which stress is seen to arise from how we appraise the pressures we face), and so psychology began to play a part, as it was recognized that it is not simply a matter of the mechanistic movement of forces, as occurs in engineering, but that there is also a significant cognitive or perceptual dimension to stress. To a limited extent this has taken account of social factors but, at best, what has developed has been a social psychology model, rather than a sociological one (see Butt's comments above about the individualism inherent in social psychology). That is, where social factors have been considered at all, they have been seen as simply contextual matters, rather than active factors in their own right. Individualization, with its tendency towards pathology and a medical model, has stood in the way of the development of a broader focus. We now, however, need to move beyond this in order to develop an enriched level of understanding to switch our focus from the narrow to the broad in order to develop a more holistic picture. In this way, we will have a greater understanding of where and how to intervene without falling into the trap of assuming that intervening at an individual level ('treatment') is necessarily the best approach.

Conclusion

Stress is a very personal experience. To find oneself in a situation where the pressures seem overwhelming and there is considerable doubt about being able to cope is to find oneself in a situation that is deeply and intimately personal. To understand stress therefore involves understanding elements of the psychology of the individual. There can be no doubt, then, that a focus on the individual is an important part of making sense of stress. However, my argument here has been that, while individual issues are an important part, they are only one part of a much more complex whole. A more holistic picture needs to include social and organizational factors—and the organizational factors need to encompass strategic as well as operational concerns. Without a consideration of these wider issues, we will be left with a very partial and distorted picture—and one that is dangerously misleading, in so far as it places major emphasis on the individual at the risk of pathologizing him or her, while leaving wider social and organizational processes unexplored.

Birch and Paul (2003) describe an Australian study of workplace stress based on a survey of over 10,000 participants. They raise a very important point when they comment on potential solutions to the problem of stress:

> Respondents were asked what they thought were solutions to stress. The main response
> was better management or more communication and consultation (53 per cent), then

came more staff and resources (30 per cent), followed by lighter workload and less monitoring (16 per cent), and better organisation of work (14 per cent). The majority were of the view that the answer to stress at work is in the workplace. Only 2.2 per cent of respondents nominated stress management programmes or courses as the answer to stress. It is the causes rather than the symptoms that need to be addressed. (pp. 105–6)

The message of this study chimes well with the argument I have been putting forward in this chapter: we need to look beyond the individual if we are to develop a realistic and helpful picture of the challenges involved in workplace stress. If we are to take seriously the challenges of promoting workplace well-being as a way of humanizing the workplace for the benefit of all concerned, then we need to make sure that we adopt a psychosocial perspective on well-being in general and stress prevention in particular.

References

Baldwin, T. (2004). *Maurice Merleau-Ponty: Basic Writings*. London: Routledge.

Bauman, Z. (2001). *The Individualized Society*. Cambridge: Polity.

Beck, U. (1992). *Risk Society*, trans. Mark Ritter. London: Sage.

Birch, C. and Paul, D. (2003). *Life and Work: Challenging Economic Man*. Sydney: UNSW Press.

Blumer, H. (1969). *Symbolic Interactionism*. Englewood Cliffs, NJ: Prentice-Hall.

Bolton, S.C. (ed.) (2007). *Dimensions of Dignity at Work*. London: Butterworth-Heinemann.

Bunting, M. (2004). *Willing Slaves: How the Overwork Culture is Ruining Our Lives*. London: HarperCollins.

Butt, T. (2004). *Understanding People*. Basingstoke: Palgrave Macmillan.

Clutterbuck, D. (2003). *Managing Work–Life Balance: A Guide for HR in Achieving Organisational and Individual Change*. London: Chartered Institute of Personnel and Development.

Cranwell-Ward, A. and Abbey, J. (2005). *Organizational Stress*. Basingstoke: Palgrave Macmillan.

DPP (Developing Patient Partnerships) (2006). *Stress and Well-being 2006: Report on New Research into Knowledge of Stress and Attitudes Towards It in the UK*. London: Developing Patient Partnerships.

Durkheim, E. (1912). *The Elementary Forms of Religious Life*, trans. C. Cosman. Oxford: Oxford World's Classics.

Earnshaw, J. and Cooper, C. (1996). *Stress and Employer Liability*. London: Institute of Personnel and Development.

Furnham, A. and Taylor, J. (2004). *The Dark Side of Behaviour at Work: Understanding and Avoiding Employees Leaving, Thieving and Deceiving*. Basingstoke: Palgrave Macmillan.

Holmes, T.H. and Rahe, R.H. (1967). The social readjustment scale. *Journal of Psychosomatic Research*, 11, 213–18.

Johnson, G. and Scholes, K. (2002). *Exploring Corporate Strategy*, 6th edn. London: Prentice-Hall.

Korcszynski, M. (2007). HRM and the menu society: The fetishisation of individual choice at work. In S.C. Bolton and M. Houlihan (eds), *Searching for the Human in Human Resource Management*. Basingstoke: Palgrave Macmillan.

Patmore, A. (2006). *The Truth About Stress*. London: Atlantic Books.

Ryan, W. (1988). *Blaming the Victim*, 2nd edn. New York: Random House.

Selye, H. (1956). *The Stress of Life*. New York: McGraw-Hill.

Shotter, J. (1993). *Cultural Politics of Everyday Life*. Buckingham: Open University Press.

Sutherland, V. J. and Cooper, C. (2000). *Strategic Stress Management: An Organizational Approach*. London: Macmillan.

Thompson, N. (2003). *Promoting Equality: Challenging Discrimination and Oppression*, 2nd edn. Basingstoke: Palgrave Macmillan.

Thompson, N. (2010). *Theorizing Social Work Practice*. Basingstoke: Palgrave Macmillan.

Thompson, N. and Bates, J. (eds) (2009). *Promoting Workplace Well-being*. Basingstoke: Palgrave Macmillan.

Thompson, N., Murphy, M., and Stradling, S. (1994). *Dealing with Stress*. Basingstoke: Macmillan.

Chapter 3

Compassion in healthcare—the missing dimension of healthcare reform?

Robin Youngson

Introduction

Robin Youngson is a UK-trained anaesthetist and clinical leader, working in New Zealand, who is leading an international campaign to strengthen humanity and compassion in healthcare. He is the founder of the Centre for Compassion in Healthcare (www.compassioninhealthcare.org).

His campaign to rehumanize healthcare was triggered by the experience of seeing his 18-year-old daughter suffering in hospital after a serious road accident. In his quest to understand how hospital services and individual practitioners could so neglect the basic human needs of patients, he has come full circle to consider how health professionals themselves experience a lack of compassion from the system that employs them. It seems that the emotional experience of patients and of health professionals is closely linked. The ultimate answer to rehumanizing healthcare and strengthening compassion, he believes, lies in the support and nurturing of health professionals.

Robin tells a deeply personal story of how his own beliefs and practice were influenced by the search for answers about the nature of compassion. His early days of professional practice were brutal and dehumanizing, leading him to adopt survival strategies of distancing and clinical detachment. But the story of his return to humanity is an inspiring example of how practitioners can heal themselves, take off their armour, and rediscover the joy of serving patients with open-hearted compassion. A supportive environment is needed to foster this kind of healing and Robin develops a model to show the integration of three important elements in the rehumanizing of healthcare:

- the development of inner resources, such as empathy and non-judgement;
- strategies to strengthen our sense of human togetherness;
- the creation of a sense of place where people find a renewed sense of shared identity and purpose.

The integration of these elements can create a community of healing that restores compassion for both practitioners and patients.

As healthcare heads into deepening crisis with workforce shortages and funding cutbacks, the tendency of governments is to impose structural reform. Robin suggests a different perspective on how we can sustain healthcare services—a renewed focus on humanity and compassion.

This is his story.

A defining moment

In any campaign to change a system there comes a defining moment when personal commitment becomes absolute. Choice is removed. That moment came to me on witnessing the plight of my 18-year-old daughter Chloe, tied to a hospital bed in traction for a broken neck. She was flat on her back, her head was completely immobilized so that she could see only the ceiling. She was unable to see people who came into her room, she couldn't see out of the window, she couldn't see a television or read a book. To sensory deprivation was added gradual starvation. There was no system to ensure that my daughter would receive adequate food—a critical component of her healing and recovery. Although she had the use of her limbs, she was unable to feed or toilet herself. For a day or two, this might be a tolerable state of affairs. Her sentence was three months.

In the beginning we imagined this neglect was a simple oversight in a busy public hospital with the usual chronic shortage of staff. However, annoyance turned to disbelief and anger when it became apparent that the hospital system was incapable of responding to these simple human needs.

There was no system to respond to the disability needs of hospital inpatients, nor was it anyone's job to ensure that patients actually received good nutrition on a daily basis, on a busy acute ward. The potential clinical consequences of these failures were severe depression, malnutrition, delayed healing, and the requirement for prolonged rehabilitation. I had worked in this hospital as a senior clinician and leader and I had extensive networks of influence. But no amount of pleading, persuasion, or anger would overcome the fact that there was a systemic failure to meet these needs and that the culture of the hospital was allowing it to happen.

In the event, Chloe walked unaided out of the hospital seven days after being released from her bonds. That she did so was a testament to her personal courage and the support of family and friends. I designed and built all of her disability and communication aids. My wife, Meredith, attended the hospital every one of the hundred days that Chloe was in hospital and ensured that she had tasty and nutritious food. We spent more than $1,000 on hospital car parking charges. The impact on the whole family was profound. But for the patients whose families did not have the privilege or resources to provide this kind of support, we were very concerned.

In general, the standard of clinical care was excellent and we are deeply grateful that our daughter was able to heal from her injuries with the dedicated care of many professionals. However, the neglect of her basic human needs she experienced can only be described as callous.

I wish Chloe's experience was an isolated case, but it's not. Ever since I began at medical school in 1980 I have been profoundly concerned about the experience of patients within the system. I have campaigned for patient-centred care, I have taught communication skills to health professionals, run workshops on humanity and compassion, and provided support for our vulnerable junior staff. In every workshop I have ever run, the participants tell me that my daughter's experience is typical of what they see every day. In 25 years of practice I have yet to find a hospital system that fully responds to the basic human needs of its patients.

And yet, within this uncaring system we found remarkable individuals whose compassion moved us profoundly. I am still undone by the memory of one act of kindness we witnessed on the first day of Chloe's long hospital stay.

Chloe made many trips within the hospital on the day of her accident: from the resuscitation room to the CT scanner; back to the trauma unit; off to the MRI scanner; transfer to the operating theatre; back to ICU. As parents we followed our daughter in these journeys and witnessed the loving care of a transit nurse. He came wonderfully prepared and thoughtful about Chloe's potential needs, with a whole kit of drugs including a generous supply of morphine.

At the junction between two hospital buildings, there is a join in the floor. Mindful of Chloe's broken neck, this wonderful nurse stopped the trolley and carefully lifted each wheel over the join in the floor to prevent any painful jolting of her injuries. Compassion is revealed in the smallest of acts.

To bewildered and frightened parents he was a trusted guide in a foreign land. He did not give us directions but took us by the hand to the places we needed to find. As the months went by, we met this nurse from time to time. He would mysteriously appear to offer wise counsel and loving concern at the times when Chloe was most distressed.

Few hospital patients ever remember what was said to them, or what was done, but the emotional experience is lived for a lifetime. The compassion and kindness of this nurse will live in our hearts forever.

What was it that sustained the humanity of this wonderful nurse when so many around him had retreated to coldly efficient practice? Conversely, how could so many health professionals witness so much suffering and yet fail to respond? The problem seems to exist at two levels. In the experience of Chloe, most of the failings were not the fault of individuals but were the consequences of gaps in the system.

But there is also the failure of individual practitioners to respond with simple measures to relieve distress, even when all the necessary resources are present. I doubt there is a more distressing experience for a health professional than seeing a loved one in excruciating pain within a system with the resources to rapidly treat that pain, but where no one is willing to take responsibility for the necessary steps. One day we watched Chloe lie for four hours in severe pain and distress as I called every professional I could think of to respond to the situation. The drug required to relieve her pain was visible to me through the glass window of the locked medication store.

Later in this chapter, I explore the professional and organizational factors that reinforce this sense of helplessness and which inhibit otherwise caring individuals from responding to distress.

Rehumanizing the role of health professionals

Personal stories can give us clues about strategies for renewing the roles of health professionals who are heading for burnout. Such a story was related by a colleague in an unexpected encounter in the hospital corridor. Mary rushed up to me and touched my arm as she said, 'Robin, there's something I must tell you!' Her story was about re-finding the heart of practice.

Mary, one of our senior clinical leaders, had some months earlier attended a workshop I facilitated on compassion and caring. The seeds of change had been sown but it took a particular encounter on the ward for the real learning to occur. Mary told me she had been asked to review the care of a frail old lady with multiple medical problems and partial blindness. When she began her assessment, she noticed the patient was distressed. She paused and asked if there was something that she could do to help. Her patient hesitatingly told her that she was extremely worried about some circumstance at home and she urgently needed to use the phone.

'Did you ask the ward nurses?' queried Mary.

'Yes,' said the old lady. 'I have asked every day to use the cordless phone but they keep telling me it's only for staff use, and I should use the patients' card phone down the corridor.' Her lips quivered and she shrugged her shoulders, helplessly.

'I can't use that phone, you see. I'm almost blind.'

Mary told me that the situation suddenly reminded her of our workshop discussion about simple acts of kindness. In that instant, she decided to respond. Excusing herself, Mary hurried to the hospital shop and purchased a phone card.Returning to the ward, she asked the old lady, 'Who is it that you need to call? I'll give you a hand.'

Taking her by the hand, Mary led the patient to the phone and helped her make the connection. The little old lady cried. This was the first time in two weeks that anyone in the hospital had listened to her personal concerns.

We can only imagine what process of healing began for the patient that day. Her heart failure and angina began to improve. It was a turning point in her hospital care.

Mary reflected on this event during the day and talked about it at home. She came to realize that this simple act of kindness was the single most satisfying thing she had done at work for a long time. Lately she had been feeling tired and stressed and wondered if she was heading for burnout. By the next morning, Mary had reconceptualized her professional role. She had always regarded herself as a clinical expert. Hence forth, she would be a caring human being first and an expert second. Each day, she looked for an opportunity to perform an unexpected act of kindness. As she told me this story, her eyes lit up and her face became animated.

'It's like I have a new job,' she said.

I cannot tell that story without being profoundly moved. We could fill this entire book with the themes and meanings of that brief encounter. At the heart of the story lies the tension between our models of impersonal, institutionalized care and the desire for the healing that brings people into the health professions. This healing is needed as much by the practitioners as those receiving care.

This story has such power for us because we all instinctively sense that health services have somehow lost a human dimension. This loss is a source of suffering for professionals, patients, and clients, and their families. When we witness the magical moments of human connection, they tug at our heartstrings and make us long for a more humane and compassionate system. Compassion is a source of renewable energy

(Maben et al., 2010; Stickley and Freshwater, 2002; Firth-Cozens and Cornwell, 2009). It sustains both the giver and the receiver and is the source of healing.

A rehumanized healthcare system must take account of the emotional, psychological, social, cultural, environmental (Metcalfe et al., 2009), and spiritual (Sulmasy, 2002; Newell 2005) dimensions of health and well-being. We could learn from indigenous people, like the Maori people of New Zealand, who describe 'Te Whare Tapa Wha,' the four cornerstones of health (Durie, 2001). They include the physical domain (*taha tinana*), the mental (*taha hinengaro*), the social/emotional (*taha whanau*), and spiritual (*taha wairua*) domains.

So I'd like to share with you my own personal journey from a role as a technical expert back to a caring and compassionate practitioner. My practice has never been more joyful or satisfying. I began my professional journey far distant from these kinds of understandings. I was an engineer first, then trained in medicine, then specialized in anaesthetics—one of the most technical branches of medicine. I became very good at clinical detachment. It's been a long journey back to my humanity.

Finally, I have some conclusions about how we might create an integrated approach to the rehumanizing of health services and other communities of caring.

A personal journey of healing

My greatest teacher was an 85-year-old patient called Jessie. She needed urgent surgery for bowel cancer but I was deeply afraid to anaesthetize her because I thought she would die on the operating table. She had the most appalling catalogue of medical complaints, including hemiplegia and severe heart disease.

On the eve of surgery, she responded compassionately to my fear and vulnerability and declared that I was 'looking much too worried about giving her anaesthetic.' She became the one doing the caring. She thought I needed cheering up so she told me a rude joke:

'What's this?' she asked, holding an unsteady finger up to her lips and blowing a wet-sounding raspberry.

'I have no idea,' I shrugged, feeling bewildered at this strange turn of events.

'It's a fart trying to get past a g-string!' she announced with great glee!

All semblance of the proper doctor–patient relationship went straight out of the window. When we had both stopped laughing we began to build a different kind of relationship. To my surprise, I slept well that night. The next day, Jessie had a stormy time in surgery and narrowly survived several anaesthetic crises. I went to visit her on the post-op ward.

'I prayed for you,' she said. 'I prayed that you would survive my anaesthetic, and you did!'

Jessie had profound lessons for me, but it would take me many years to realize their full potential. She taught me that the relationship between doctors and their patients is a two-way street; caring and compassion can flow in both directions. She allowed me to understand that shared humanity was a more secure foundation for practice than any amount of technical expertise. She demonstrated the power of laughter to ease fear and make a connection. And she showed how choosing an attitude can transform those around you.

As I write these words, I am sitting in my hospital on a Tuesday afternoon, on duty for calls to the maternity unit. I am the on-call anaesthetist doing epidurals for pain relief in labour and providing anaesthesia for emergency Caesarean sections or other medical procedures.

I work a 24-hour shift. Childbirth is not an office-hours business. Sometimes I'm called out several times in the night, becoming fatigued and sleep deprived. In those circumstances, it's only natural to feel somewhat grumpy and sorry for yourself. I used to carry my grumpiness into work with me and be intolerant of frustrations, delays, or missing equipment. I didn't always experience the friendliest of receptions when I entered the labour room. Sometimes it felt like I was the enemy, the 'wicked' doctor come to intervene in childbirth when the plan was for a natural process with no drugs and no technology. It was an uphill struggle to find the necessary equipment, to ask the midwife to get the mother positioned for the epidural, and to communicate instructions. Sometimes the epidural didn't work well and I'd be called out of bed again. I was overwhelmed with negative thoughts, tired, and grumpy.

One night, driving into the hospital for the third or fourth time, feeling quite sorry for myself, I suddenly felt ashamed. If Jessie could choose a positive attitude in her dire circumstance, then what right did I have to be grumpy?

I chose to put different thoughts in my head. Now, when I'm called out in the middle of the night I think about the extraordinary privilege of being invited to take part in an intimate and life-changing event. I take great care with the spirit and presence I bring into the room. I enter the room with gentleness, quietness, and compassion. I notice the effect this has on the mother in reducing fear and distress. I greet and acknowledge the other people in the room. I ask after the midwife, enquire whether she has been busy or had any sleep. I do the epidural with the minimum of fuss and then witness the miracle of pain relief. It is a joyous experience. I don't care how tired I am. I go home with love and joy in my heart.

How amazingly the world changed when I chose to have a different attitude! Now I feel like an honoured visitor. I am greeted warmly by the midwives. I have the sense that my praises have been sung to the mother even before I step into the labour room. An extra special effort will be made to anticipate what I need to make preparation for the procedure. I find that the pain relief is much more effective and the rate of complications is greatly reduced.

For most of my career, I considered the problem of the relationship with midwives as a problem 'out there'. My more recent experience leads me to believe that the problem and certainly the solution existed in my own head. The only person who changed was me. But the consequence of that was a remarkable change in my whole world experience.

Sometimes you have to change 'me' to change the world.

As my practice deepened I began to reflect on my role, how I might best serve my patients, and where I might find the sources of the deepest satisfaction and joy. I came to realize that for much of my career, my identity and self-esteem were wrapped up in being a highly trained technical expert. I was always friendly and helpful but I was certainly the person in charge of the agenda. If my patients brought up other concerns or questions, beyond the scope of my technical expertise, I was skilled at diverting them back onto safer ground. Over time, I have gradually reconceptualized my role as that of a caring human being first, and an expert second. That enabled me to be much more humble and respectful, to listen patiently, to form more trusting relationships with my patients, and to bring much greater compassion and humanity to the relationship. I began to take great pleasure in helping patients in whatever way I could, regardless of whether it related to my specific technical role as an anaesthetic specialist.

One day, I decided that I would no longer have 'difficult' patients. I decided that difficult patients didn't exist 'out there' but were a consequence of my attitudes or judgement, an internal problem. I decided that if a patient continued to make demands, or to break rules, or otherwise be disruptive, it was a matter of my failing to understand or meet some need. I owned the problem as my own, rather than projecting it out onto the patient.

When I changed my attitude, I noticed an immediate effect. Often the patients were surprised or taken aback. They were quite unused to doctors treating them with respect. I found it was easy to negotiate solutions for particular problems with a bit of give-and-take on both sides. I often have to be an advocate for the patient but it is usually a small matter of negotiating agreement with the rest of the staff. Quite suddenly I found I didn't have difficult patients any more. This was definitely an improvement in the quality of my working day! But paradoxically, the only person who changed was me.

I was so encouraged with the positive results of this experiment that I decided to extend it to all my patients. I decided to take the attitude that no patient of mine ever made unreasonable demands and I would simply do my best to respond to every matter brought to my attention. I would be attentive, I would try not to judge, I would be careful in the use of power, I would let the patient set the agenda, and I would continually seek permission and approval for the process we were following together.

My colleagues thought I was completely mad. It was obvious to them that I would soon be overwhelmed, exhausted, and burnt out. In their experience, patients continually made demands that couldn't be met and they had to employ a variety of means to defend themselves against this unreasonable onslaught.

My experience was of completely the opposite effect. The demands of my patients grew less, not more. In this paradox lies a clue to the source of abundance.

The key insight is that there is a difference between fixing, helping, and serving. I finally understood the distinction when I read a wonderful paper by Rachel Remen, 'In the service of life' (Remen 1996). Fixing is often the appropriate course of action for an acute condition or injury, or where chronic disability can be reversed through technology such as hip-joint replacement. Fixing puts the expert in charge, but that's fine for the right kind of problem. The patient has a short-term contract: I put myself in your hands for the sake of achieving this specific improvement. It's a transactional relationship.

Of course, many of the chronic problems we see don't have a technical solution and they can't be fixed. While on the surface 'helping' seems a laudable approach, we should be mindful of the resulting power relationship. The helper is always in a position of power over the person being helped. It's a dependent relationship that takes power away from patients. They take less responsibility for their own health and well-being because it's the doctor's job to fix the problem.

As long as the doctor is stuck in the 'helper' mode, demand will be unrelenting. In the end, chronically helping and rescuing diminishes our patients; it makes them less capable of dealing with their own life problems.

So why is my experience different? I choose to serve my patients on their own terms. You can tell when someone is truly being served because you witness personal growth. The person being served takes greater responsibility for their own health and well-being. Their capacity for dealing with life's challenges is enhanced by your coaching and support. The relationship is one of deep mutual respect, honesty, and openness. In this circumstance, no patient makes unreasonable demands. The workload for the doctor decreases not increases. However, the joy and satisfaction in work is greatly enhanced. It become a privilege to be invited to participate in intimate life events and to witness the extraordinary courage and generosity of ordinary people as they struggle with this thing called 'life'. I certainly take delight in seeing their growing capacity for effective and wise responses to life's challenges.

Now I have learned to be still and to listen. Sometimes, quiet presence without anxiety is the most profound intervention. Brokenness is part of the human condition. We do not need to fix it or hide it, just be present and share our common experience of humanity.

To step aside from the expert role and to bring the quality of compassionate, non-anxious presence requires a deal of inner work. Humility and non-judgement are important qualities. As the inner resources are cultivated, so one develops greater mindfulness, presence, patience, gentleness, and a powerful sense of meaning and purpose. The end result is great joy, satisfaction, and increased resilience.

Challenging models of professionalism

My own long journey of learning suggests to me that we need to challenge existing models of professionalism. The Western model rests on foundations of a biomedical approach, rational detachment, and objectivity. There is also a widespread belief that emotional attachment to patients is hazardous to professional well-being and that clinical detachment is a necessary defence when witnessing the suffering of patients.

Research shows that medical students lose the ability to empathize with their patients during clinical training and instead identify with the hero model of the medical practitioner. They are 'drawn to doctors whom they have idealized as healthy, invulnerable, authoritative, skilled and effective individuals who possess powerful and still somewhat mysterious knowledge and skills' (Shapiro, 2008).

We have much to learn from other cultures. Contrary to prevailing Western beliefs, the experience of all who empathize deeply with their patients and bring open-hearted compassion to their work is that they increase their store of love—provided that they have a supportive environment that allows them to develop their inner resources. Empathy, compassion, and loving kindness have a biological basis. The regular focus on compassion and mindfulness strengthens those parts of the brain associated with positive emotions (Lutz et al., 2008) and diminishes the risk of burnout and compassion fatigue (Krasner et al., 2009; Gilbert and Procter, 2006).

In 'Walking a mile in their patients' shoes', Shapiro writes a comprehensive review of the psychological and emotional responses to the traumas of clinical training and practice and shows how a more humanistic approach can strengthen empathy and the capacity for compassionate caring (Shapiro, 2008). It should be compulsory reading for every professional body reviewing models of professionalism and codes of practice.

The reintegration of humane and compassionate practice

While the development of our inner resources for compassion and caring is essential, we cannot do this without support. There is a broader set of human needs (Todres et al., 2009) that must be met to create sustainable communities of caring, including a need for 'togetherness' and a 'sense of place'. When these come together, the heart is filled. (See Figure 3.1.)

However, there are a powerful set of forces in our modern health services that are causing a disintegration of humane and compassionate caring.

◆ The disease focus, reductionism, and super-specialization all deny our humanity and hinder the development of our inner resources for caring, leaving us feeling powerless and overwhelmed (Cole and Carlin, 2009).

◆ The traumatization of young professionals in their training and early practice (National Patient Safety Foundation, 2009), widespread bullying in healthcare (Johnson, 2009), and unresolved emotional responses to human suffering and loss, lead to distancing and isolation rather than trusting relationships (Shapiro, 2008).

◆ The cold clinical environment, the imposition of alien corporate cultures and values, and the lack of attention to spiritual values mean that we lose the sense of place, of our shared identity and purpose. We suffer a dislocation and loss of meaning in our work. (See Figure 3.2.)

But when we create a safe and healthy environment, a different set of qualities can begin to flourish.

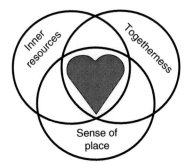

Fig. 3.1 Elements of a sustainable community of caring.

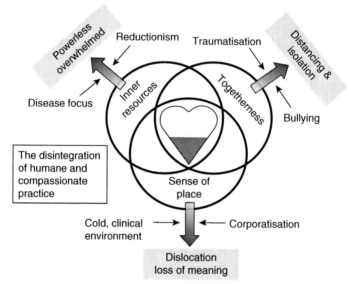

Fig. 3.2 The disintegration of humane and compassionate practice.

We need to act fearlessly against bullying. We need to create a humane and supportive work environment so that our caregivers can develop the inner resources for compassionate caring (Kearney et al., 2009; Epstein, 1999; Krasner et al., 2009; Gilbert and Procter, 2006). Caregivers need to feel safe enough to take off the 'armour' of clinical detachment and bring greater humanity to their work (Youngson, 2010). When we make mistakes, we need to have the courage to apologize, to be honest, and to make amends (Bismark and Paterson, 2005). We need to encourage mutual support and shared learning among our different professional groups and between caregivers, patients, and their families. When we do all these things, we create a sense of togetherness.

We need to build warm and welcoming places of healing, not cold, clinical environments. Our hospitals and clinics need to relate to the natural environment in a way that signals a concern with the health of future generations and the healing of the present. We must strengthen our connections to the communities we serve and build a powerful sense of shared identity and meaning. And we should allow our spiritual side to find expression (Youngson, 2007).

There is a deep congruence in the values expressed through these many changes. When we do all these things, the heart begins to fill again. (Figure 3.3.)

I have one final story from New Zealand. I was involved for many years in the development of a small community hospital to serve an underprivileged population in west Auckland. Before the new Waitakere Hospital was opened a sacred ceremony took place in the cold hours before dawn, attending to spiritual values that span two cultures. Four hundred hospital staff and community members gathered at 5.00 a.m. to partake in a blessing ceremony. Led by Maori elders, chanting prayers and incantations, the long file of people entered every room of the new building touching the walls

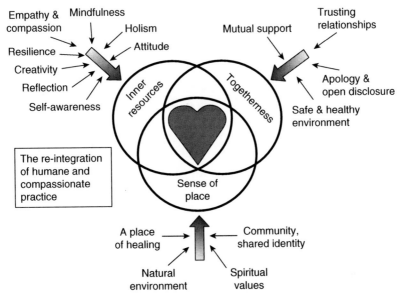

Empathy & compassion
Mindfulness
Holism
Attitude
Resilience
Creativity
Reflection
Self-awareness
Inner resources
Togetherness
Mutual support
Trusting relationships
Apology & open disclosure
Safe & healthy environment
The re-integration of humane and compassionate practice
Sense of place
A place of healing
Community, shared identity
Natural environment
Spiritual values

Fig. 3.3 The reintegration of humane and compassionate practice.

and fittings to add the warmth of their human spirit to the cold walls. The procession took two hours and was concluded with a feast as the sun rose. In turn, this sacred building touches all who enter it.

References

Bismark, M. and Paterson, R. (2005). 'Doing the right thing' after an adverse event. *New Zealand Medical Journal*, **118**, 1219–23.

Cole, T. and Carlin, N. (2009). The suffering of physicians. *The Lancet*, **374**, 1414–15.

Durie, M. (2001). *Mauri Ora: The Dynamics of Maori Health*. Oxford: Oxford University Press.

Epstein, R. (1999). Mindful practice. *Journal of the American Medical Association*, **282**(9), 833–9.

Firth-Cozens, J. and Cornwell, J. (2009). *The point of care: Enabling compassionate care in acute hospital settings*. Report of the King's Fund available at: http://www.kingsfund.org.uk/document.rm?id=8295 (accessed 29 May 2010).

Gilbert, P. and Procter, S. (2006). Compassionate mind training for people with high shame and self-criticism: Overview and pilot study of a group therapy approach. *Clinical Psychology and Psychotherapy*, **13**, 353–79.

Johnson, S.L. (2009). International perspectives on workplace bullying among nurses: a review. *International Nursing Review*, **56**, 34–40.

Kearney, M., Weininger, R., Vachon, M., et al. (2009). Self-care of physicians at the end of life: 'Being connected . . . a key to my survival'. *Journal of the American Medical Association*, **301**(11), 1155–64.

Krasner, M.S., Epstein, R.M., Beckman, H., et al. (2009). Association of an Educational Program in Mindful Communication with Burnout, Empathy, and Attitudes Among Primary Care Physicians. *Journal of the American Medical Association*, **302**(12), 1284–93.

Lutz, A., Brefczynski-Lewis, J., Johnstone, T., and Davidson, R.J. (2008). Regulation of the neural circuitry of emotion by compassion meditation: Effects of meditative expertise. *PLoS ONE*, **3**(3), e1897.

Maben, J., Cornwell, J., and Sweeney, S. (2010). In praise of compassion. *Journal of Research in Nursing*, **15**(1), 9–13.

Metcalfe, S., Woodward, A., McMillan, A., et al. (2009). Why New Zealand must rapidly halve its greenhouse gas emissions. *New Zealand Medical Journal*, **122**(1304), 72–95.

National Patient Safety Foundation (2009). *Disrespectful and abusive behaviour: The 'hidden curriculum' of medical school. Focus on patient safety—a newsletter of the NPSF 2009*; vol. 12, no. 1. Available at: http://npsf.org/paf/npsfp/fo/pdf/Focus_Volume_12_%20Issue_1.pdf (accessed 29 May 2010).

Newell, C. (2005). Disability, spirituality and pastoral care. *New Zealand Journal of Disability Studies*, **11**, 103–19.

Remen, R. (1996). In the service of life. *Noetic Sciences Review*, **37**, 24–5.

Shapiro, J. (2008). Walking a mile in their patients' shoes: empathy and othering in medical students' education. *Philosophy, Ethics, and Humanities in Medicine*, **3**, 10–20.

Stickley, T. and Freshwater, D. (2002). The art of loving and the therapeutic relationship. *Nursing Inquiry*, **9**(4), 250–6.

Sulmasy, D. (2002). A biopsychosocial-spiritual model for the care of patients at the end of life. *The Gerontologist*, **42** (special issue iii), 24–33.

Todres, L., Galvin, K., and Dahlberg, K. (2007). Lifeworld-led healthcare: Revisiting a humanising philosophy that integrates emerging trends. *Medicine, Health Care and Philosophy*, **10**(1), 53–63.

Todres, L., Galvin, K., and Holloway, I. (2009). The humanization of healthcare: A value framework for qualitative research. *International Journal of Qualitative Studies on Health and Well-being*, **4**(2), 68–77.

Youngson, R. (2007). *The organisational domain of people centred care*. Report. Technical paper for the World Health Organization in the launch of 'People at the Centre of Health Care: Harmonising Mind and Body, People and Systems', Tokyo, 25 Nov. Available at: http://www.wpro.who.int/sites/pci/publications.htm (accessed 29 May 2010).

Youngson, R. (2010). Taking off the armor. *Illness, Crisis & Loss*, **18**(1), 79–82.

Chapter 4

Revisiting empathic engagement: countering compassion fatigue with 'Exquisite Empathy'

Radhule Weininger and Michael Kearney

It is recognized that those working in end-of-life care are at risk for Compassion Fatigue and Burnout. While being seen as valuable clinical assets, emotional openness and empathic availability are frequently characterized as a liability to the clinician and a more distant professional demeanor as being protective. Recent research, however, challenges these assumptions and suggests that there is a particular form of empathic engagement that can be both protective and replenishing. This has been called 'Exquisite Empathy'.
(Harrison and Westwood, 2009)

In this chapter the concept of 'Exquisite Empathy' will be explored. We will examine how, by participating in a programme designed to enhance clinician self-awareness, it is possible to practise empathic engagement in a way that is mutually regenerative for patient and clinician. It is proposed that self-awareness-based empathic engagement allows clinicians to be simultaneously heartfelt and protected in their clinical encounters.

Introduction

I would like to start this chapter by sharing my personal story as a clinician faced with the challenge of finding a model of self-care that allowed me to be emotionally protected in work situations and at the same time present for my patients, without getting hardened or burned out. For a long time I had felt a silent dissonance underlying my experience as a therapist, as a leader of groups for people with AIDS, and as a physician. My training emphasized the need to keep strict boundaries and distance;

that becoming too close and too 'loving' with patients would make me 'less professional' as a clinician. I was also taught that less distant behaviour would take a personal toll and leave me depleted and worn out. My own heart as well as my Buddhist training in Loving Kindness and compassion told me otherwise and led me to doubt these commonly held assumptions. I shared these conflicting feelings with my co-author Michael Kearney, a palliative care physician, in the context of our planning to do some teaching together about professional relationships and empathy to groups of clinicians working in end-of-life care.

One evening the discussion took a new turn. After a meditation group I had been leading ended, a man called Richard Harrison introduced himself to me. Richard was a counselling psychologist from the University of British Columbia in Vancouver, Canada, now working in the University of California in Santa Barbara. In the discussion that followed I learned that he had made a curious discovery in his dissertation research. One of his findings was that, under certain favourable conditions, a group of exemplary trauma therapists, all of whom had worked for a long time in their field, did not feel, as might have been expected, depleted, and traumatized by their work with abused patients. Rather they described how they felt replenished by doing meaningful and heartfelt work. Richard and his colleague Marvin Westwood identified a number of protective practices that appeared to explain this. One of these was a certain type of empathic engagement, which they called 'Exquisite Empathy'. These findings challenged the prevailing wisdom that being empathic makes the clinician more vulnerable in the therapeutic encounter (Figley, 1995). Among other protective practices identified by Richard and his colleague were that these therapists had developed ways of countering isolation, and embracing complexity and holistic self-care. What particularly caught my attention was that a common theme underlying all these practices appeared to be clinician self-awareness.

Interestingly, at just this time I was invited to participate as a co-author on an article on the self-care of physicians working in end-of-life care. Recognizing the unique contribution that Richard's findings brought to this discussion I suggested that he might also come onboard as co-author, which he did. The article was published in the *Journal of the American Medical Association* in March 2009 (Kearney et al., 2009).

Even though Richard Harrison's findings are only valid for a relatively small study population, they seem to speak to a larger philosophical, socio-political, and ethical conundrum: the tendency for clinicians to categorize, objectify, and therefore separate themselves from their patients, which appears to be embedded in wider cultural, philosophical, and economic principles of our society. My own view, based on 20 years of clinical practice, is that, rather than being protective, a standoffish and distant professional demeanour may actually be damaging for both the patient and the clinician. Perhaps, rather than finding protection in distancing, what we need both individually and collectively, in this social climate that seems to be becoming colder, with fear seeping in through the cracks of our social and political fabric, is a new way of relating. Is it possible to find a way of being open, loving, and sensitized in our relations with others, while at the same time being protected? If so, such a new way of relating would have to strike a delicate balance between caring for ourselves and being open to the world we encounter.

Burnout

Burnout may result from stresses that arise from the clinician's interaction with their work environment, or from the mismatch between corporate values and those of the individual (Maslach et al., 2001). As one medical oncologist put it, 'The stuff that burns me out has nothing to do with loss... It's fighting with insurance companies...' (Kearney et al., 2009, p. 1156). Other examples of the 'stuff' of burnout might include too much work, too many long days, having to attend to too many people in too short of time, too little time to recuperate, and too little support from others. Clinicians suffering from burnout might experience overwhelming physical and emotional exhaustion, feelings of cynicism and detachment from their job, coupled with a sense of ineffectiveness and a lack of accomplishment (Maslach and Leiter, 2008). Other symptoms of burnout that have been reported include poor judgement, over-identification or over-involvement, boundary violations, perfectionism and rigidity, interpersonal conflicts, addictive behaviours, frequent illnesses that include headaches and gastrointestinal disturbances, and immune system impairment (Maslach et al., 2001). Clinicians who burn out may even question the meaning of their lives and their prior religious beliefs (Vachon, 2010).

Compassion fatigue

In contrast to burnout, 'compassion fatigue' evolves specifically from the relationship between the clinician and the patient (Figley, 1995, p7). Compassion fatigue is also described as Secondary Traumatic Stress Disorder, the hypothesis being that clinicians can be traumatized by getting too close to their patients' suffering (ibid.). In the process, a clinician's own unresolved trauma material and unconscious unresolved childhood conflicts can be stimulated (Hayes, 2004). The symptoms of compassion fatigue include those of Post-traumatic Stress Disorder (PTSD) such as increased arousal, irritability and hyper-vigilance, difficulty concentrating, re-experiencing memories of difficult clinical situations, avoidance of similar ones, intrusive thoughts, sleep problems including nightmares, social withdrawal, and even numbness or disassociation (Garfield, 1995; Wright, 2004).

In a view that has broad acceptance, the caregiver's empathy level with the traumatized individual plays a significant role in this transmission (Figley, 1995; Hojat et al., 2002). The implication here seems to be that we may be better off not giving too much, and keeping ourselves well-protected behind strict professional boundaries. Yet, we also observe the increased isolation, alienation, emotional drying-up, disenchantment and lack of enthusiasm in many clinicians. Even caring work can become drained of meaning, and begin to feel more like a business, beset with management challenges, just like all other professions. Could it be that emotional distancing as the primary strategy of professional self-protection is, in fact, actually exacerbating the very problem it is intended to help?

Exquisite Empathy

The concept of Exquisite Empathy offers another possibility. It suggests that it may be possible to give more of ourselves in our clinical encounters, if we do this in the right way, and that this could be enriching and healing for both patients and clinicians. In their paper, Harrison and Westwood report that 'most of the clinicians described how intimate empathic engagement with clients sustains them in their work' (Harrison and Westwood, 2009, p. 13). They continue:

> When therapists maintain clarity about interpersonal boundaries, when they are able to get very close without fusing or confusing the patient's story, experiences, and perspectives with their own, this exquisite kind of empathic attunement is nourishing for therapist and client alike, in part because the therapists recognize it is beneficial to the clients. Participants who engaged in Exquisite Empathy describe having been invigorated rather than depleted by their intimate professional connections with traumatized clients. (Harrison and Westwood, 2009, p. 213)

We believe that Harrison and Westwood's findings are relevant in a wide variety of clinical contexts. Indeed, one could postulate that the concept of Exquisite Empathy is relevant beyond the clinical setting for many of our human interactions.

Exquisite Empathy is described as empathic engagement that is 'discerning, highly present, sensitively attuned, well-boundaried and heartfelt' (ibid., p. 213). This is a quality of relationship that one can develop towards oneself, towards others, and towards the world. The concept of Exquisite Empathy could be seen as a contemporary psychological re-visiting of Martin Buber's idea of an 'I–Thou' relationship (Buber, 1970).

The practice of Exquisite Empathy

We need to consider how to develop, over time, the skills that will enable us to practice Exquisite Empathy in the present moment. Comparable to learning to meditate or play the violin, the successful practice of Exquisite Empathy is made possible and enhanced by developing a very particular skill set. The practice of Exquisite Empathy appears to be facilitated by clinician self-awareness (Harrison and Westwood, 2009). Clinician self-awareness, in our definition, involves four overlapping and complementary practices: the practice of self-knowledge; the practice of self-empathy; the practice of preparing the mind through Mindfulness practice; and the practice of contemplative awareness.

Self-knowledge

Following the Delphic imperative to 'Know thyself!', self-knowledge prepares the ground for clinician self-awareness. This includes becoming familiar with one's family history, one's cultural, racial, and religious history, as well as one's individual talents and challenges. Having deep insight into our background allows us to work through emotional challenges so that these will not get repressed or projected onto others. This also includes knowledge about our emotional lives, why and when we shut down, our capacity for openness, and especially, our areas of emotional reactivity.

It may be helpful for the clinician to engage in psychotherapy with a skilled psychotherapist. Within a secure and confidential therapeutic container, the clinician, now patient, finds the security to open up and to explore. Psychotherapy increases awareness, enables recognition of habitual patterns of reaction, and opens the possibility of choosing other possible responses to a given situation. It helps the clinician to better manage distress and discomfort and encourages clear thinking on how to improve communication and relationships.

Within the psychotherapeutic relationship unconscious processes can be made conscious, and distressing emotions associated with painful family histories can be worked through. In this way the unconscious phenomena of 'transference' and 'counter-transference' can be recognized and named, bringing greater insight to both patient and clinician. Transference is characterized by the unconscious redirection of feelings from one person to another, for example, from patient to clinician. Transference can be seen as a re-emergence of emotions, which originate in repressed experiences especially those from childhood. Then the clinician appearing in the patient's life can be substituted for the original object of repressed impulses. For example, it was difficult for a female patient, Sarah, who had been deeply traumatized by her father, to see her male doctor as a benign figure and allow his help, as her fear led her to *transfer* unconscious feelings of mistrust of her father onto her doctor.

Counter-transference, in contrast, addresses unconscious feelings that might arise in the clinician, stimulated through contact with the patient. Counter-transference could be seen as the inappropriate repetition in the present of a relationship that was important in a person's past. For example, a doctor, who had a complaining, self-important, and always sickly mother, and who was unaware that he was repressing feelings of frustration towards her, had trouble feeling true empathy for certain female patients, especially those with some resemblance to his mother. Awareness of his unconscious feelings and addressing them with a therapist, allowed the therapeutic relationship with such patients to be freer, healthier, and much more rewarding.

Clinical supervision, where the clinician meets regularly with another professional who possesses greater training and experience to discuss casework and professional issues, and ongoing continuing education, which helps the clinician to stay current with newly emerging treatment approaches and to deepen her/his understanding about cultural, sexual, political, and spiritual issues, are also ways of increasing clinician self-awareness.

Self-empathy

Self-empathy is a form of self-knowledge that involves being aware of the state of one's own heart. This may include noticing the degree to which we are open to affection from others and when we shut down. Self-empathy also includes noticing how critical we are ourselves, and how hard it is to accept our imperfections and mistakes with an attitude of warmth and self-acceptance, and a commitment to find a way to end that suffering in ourselves. Self-empathy is not just about self-care. It also affects the quality of our empathic connection to others; 'Self-empathy opens the way to interpersonal empathy' (Barrett-Leonard, 1997).

Certain practices from the Buddhist tradition are particularly helpful in developing self-empathy. Self-empathy is enhanced by deliberately adopting a self-compassionate attitude towards ourselves while practising Mindfulness Meditation. Sharon Salzberg writes, 'The heart of compassion is known in Buddhist teaching as the quivering of the heart in response to pain or suffering' (Salzburg, 2008). Meta or Loving-Kindness Meditation is an explicit practice of opening the heart with empathy and compassion. This practice is an effective way of balancing the presence and wisdom developed through Mindfulness Meditation. In his writings, psychologist and Buddhist teacher Jack Kornfield suggests that one needs to feel tenderness, mercy for all that arises within ourselves that is painful, confused, shameful, or frightened. He writes, 'Compassion for our own fear and shame opens us to others' (Kornfield, 2008). He continues, 'Love is our true nature, but as we have seen, it is covered over by a protective layer of fear. Even though this love is innate, the Buddhist path also uses systemic trainings to cultivate this love. They strengthen our capacity for love, compassion, joy, and peace' (ibid., p. 386).

The purpose of Meta Meditation is to actively cultivate kindness and compassion for oneself and others through mindful and heartfelt repetition of certain phrases that are traditionally used. We begin by directing love and kindness towards ourselves:

- May I be filled with love and kindness
- May I be safe and live my life with ease
- May I be well in body, heart, mind, and soul
- May I be peaceful and truly happy.

There are ways you can expand on this meditation. You can send your good wishes to your family, friends, neighbours, or to people you feel neutral about. You can also apply this meditation to people you find challenging, for example towards those to whom you feel an aversion. You may extend your well-wishing to all beings, humans and animals. Be gentle and patient with yourself as you do this. You may choose to dedicate this practice, for example, to the expansion of your heart and the well-being of others.

When practising Meta or Loving-Kindness Meditation, one needs to be careful, so that the practice stays authentic and truthful, and one does not fall into wishful thinking. Therefore, three steps are recommended. The first involves setting the intention to wish ourselves or another well. The next step involves our slowly and silently repeating those phrases of well-wishing towards ourselves and others described above, while infusing our words with feelings of good-will. This may prove to be difficult if not impossible, especially for individuals who have had neglectful or traumatic pasts, or are so hurt in their sense of self, that wishing themselves or others well turns out to be impossible. As a third step we can notice this is so and realize that we can choose to accept that is what true for us at this time.

Another Tibetan Buddhist meditation practice, 'Tonglen', describes a way of connecting with suffering, our own and that of others that can lead to a deepening sense of compassion. The practice of Tonglen can lead to a transformation in our relationship to suffering, such that we are no longer so fearful of it, and to our needing to have a less defended heart.

The practice of Tonglen begins by bringing mindful attention to another who is suffering. As we come to sense this person, our inhalation is infused with the wish to take away all the pain and fear of that person. As we exhale we send the suffering patient happiness, health, or whatever might relieve their suffering. In practising Tonglen we may notice that we are inhibited by our own fear, resistance, anger, or personal worries. In this case it may be helpful to extend the practice to ourselves. As we become aware of our particular suffering, we may keep in mind others who at this moment are having similar experiences. Then our breathing-in becomes an act of well-wishing not just for ourselves but for all the people who are caught in similar experiences of suffering, and our exhalation an act of sending out relief to both ourselves and others. The practice of Tonglen reverses the usual logic of avoiding suffering and seeking pleasure, helping us to move beyond self-preoccupation to a more compassionate and inclusive perspective (Bloom, 2000).

A final meditation practice from the Buddhist tradition that may be helpful in developing self-empathy is the practice of 'Shen-Pa', as described by Pema Chodron (Chodron, 2006). In Shen-Pa Meditation, one learns how to experience and hold the physical sensations accompanying strong emotions or thoughts. An underlying premise to this practice is that tactile sensations precede thoughts and emotions. Therefore, as we learn to recognize, face, and experience uncomfortable physical sensations, for example a tightness around the heart, and to simultaneously refrain from avoiding or fighting this, or of dissociating from it, we may begin to develop a relationship with the painful complex of which the physical sensation is a somatic expression, become intimate with it, and overcome our fear of it.

Preparing the mind

For the purpose of teaching the practice of Exquisite Empathy we differentiate three aspects of training the mind: focused awareness, mindful self-awareness, and dual-awareness. *Mindfulness Meditation* practice can be used to cultivate these three cognitive skills, which are synergistic with one another. Jon Kabat-Zinn, whose teachings derive from the Theravaden Buddhist tradition, describes Mindfulness Meditation as a process of developing careful attention to minute shifts in body, mind, emotions, and the environment, while holding a kind, non-judgemental attitude towards self and others (Kabat-Zinn, 2003).

Focused awareness is the platform from which we prepare the mind and is taken here to mean the stabilization and direction of attention. Alan Wallace, coming from the Tibetan Buddhist tradition, writes, 'From a Buddhist perspective, the untrained mind is afflicted with attention deficits and hyperactivity; it is dysfunctional. Like a wild elephant, the untamed mind can inflict enormous damage on ourselves and those around us' (Wallace, 2006). He describes the first stage of gathering the mind as directed attention. 'The sign of having reached the stage [of focussed awareness] is simply being able to place your mind on your chosen object of meditation for even a second or two' (ibid., p. 14). Wallace emphasizes the importance of deep relaxation, stabilization of the mind, and an attitude of vividness in his method of teaching mindfulness of breathing. The core practice is simply described: 'Mindfulness of breathing means settling your awareness on the sensations involved in breathing, continually returning your attention whenever your mind wanders' (ibid., pp. 6–7). While the breath is the primary touchstone, we learn to simultaneously notice and name whatever thoughts, feelings and sensations may arise. This practice, which Wallace describes as settling the mind in its natural state, enables us, over time, to allow the activities and manifestations of the mind to go by without grasping them.

Mindful self-awareness arises naturally from focused awareness and is described as a 'non-judging, respectful awareness' that enables us to witness the stream of our thoughts, physical symptoms, and feelings, and at the same time to notice when we are reacting, comparing, and evaluating. Through mindful self-awareness we learn to be with ourselves with kindness and without commentary or judgement.

Kornfield proposes using the tools of recognition, acceptance, investigation, and non-identification (R-A-I-N) to develop mindful self-awareness (Kornfield, 2008). *Recognition* refers to 'the willingness to see what is so' (ibid., p. 102). Recognition of physical sensations precedes recognition of thoughts and feelings; for example, a sensation of tightness around the heart or the sensation of a tight knot in the stomach precedes the thought that we are scared or upset. '*Acceptance* allows us to relax and open to the facts before us' (ibid., p. 102). Without acceptance and self-compassion the sudden awareness of our internal process including the multitude of sensations, feelings, and thoughts could be overwhelming and discouraging. Through *investigation* we can become aware of 'what is happening within our body, we can notice what feelings are part of this journey and look into the mind and see what thoughts and images are associated with this experience' (ibid., p. 104). As we investigate our experience without analysis, investigation, or judgement, we can learn to respect and even befriend them. *Non-identification* means to stop taking our experience so personally. When we are less attached to our experience as 'me or mine' we are freer to allow what is. 'Without identification we can respectfully care for ourselves and others yet we are no longer bound by the fears and illusions of the small sense of self' (ibid., p. 106). Non-identification may allow us to recognize the impermanent and universal nature of experience.

Developing mindful self-awareness through the practice of Mindfulness Meditation allows us to carry the skill of being present and introspective into the rest of our lives. We can then apply being mindfully present to moments of challenge, including interactions with patients, clients, neighbours, or relatives. Having a regular practice of Mindfulness Meditation allows us to carry the skill of being present and introspective into the rest of our lives.

Dual-awareness is a cognitive stance that permits the clinician to simultaneously attend to and monitor the needs of the patient and/or the work environment and his or her own subjective experience. In other words, it is the ability to be simultaneously aware of one's inner and outer experience without reactivity, or at least with the ability to be conscious of one's reactivity. In practice it means being able to notice our thoughts, feelings, bodily sensations, triggers, and reactions, while simultaneously holding our outer experience, including how we experience the person in front of us, without being drawn into or overwhelmed by that experience unwillingly.

The skill of dual-awareness takes a lot of practice and presence of mind, yet it can be learned through meditation practice and good instruction. Dual-awareness builds on the practices of focused awareness and mindful self-awareness. Through focused and mindful self-awareness we attend to and witness our experience in a non-judgemental way. As we do so we may notice moments of expanded awareness, when we are aware that we are aware of the object of our focused mindfulness, or possibly that we have just been distracted by a thought. This is dual-awareness, also sometimes referred to as 'meta-attention'. With time and practice we can deliberately choose this cognitive stance and use it to monitor the quality of our attention in meditation practice. As we become more experienced in 'shifting gears' between focused and mindful awareness and dual-awareness we can begin to bring our awareness to our inner and outer reality at the same time and use this skill in clinical and social contacts as a means of self-monitoring and self-awareness. Developing the skill of dual-awareness helps to prevent us from getting trapped in reactivity or self-preoccupation, or or from becoming over-identified with the other in the relationship, or trapped in 'tunnel vision' where we get so engaged with the other that we lose sight of the whole *gestalt* of the situation.

Dual-awareness is also being used in the field of trauma therapy as a means of countering the dissociating effects of PTSD. Babette Rothchild describes how this works: 'Developing or reconnecting with the ability for dual awareness enables the client to address a trauma while secure in the knowledge that the actual, present environment is trauma-free. It is an extremely useful tool for healing discrepancies between the experience and observing selves' (Rothchild, 2000). In other words through dual-awareness a client can be grounded in the safety of the present moment while simultaneously attending to the unsafe content associated with the trauma event. This may also have relevance in the treatment of compassion fatigue/secondary traumatization.

Contemplative awareness

Contemplative awareness is an awareness of how we as individuals are situated in a larger field of relationships. Psychologically this is sometimes referred to as the intersubjective field. Spiritually, this could be seen as a meaningful field of interconnectedness. In various religious traditions contemplative awareness could be seen as the experience of our relationship to the sacred. It includes becoming aware how we find meaning through our values, our spiritual ethics and our cosmology or philosophy of life.

Martin Buber's concept of 'I–Thou' shows great humanism and spiritual wisdom and speaks to the spiritual underpinning of relating in a heartfelt way that is rooted in contemplative awareness. In his book *I and Thou* (Buber, 1970), Buber distinguishes between two types of interpersonal relationships. In the first of these, which he calls the I–It relationship, we relate to others as objects or members of categories. In the other, in the I–Thou relationship, we relate with the entirety of our being to another whole person with an understanding of the sacredness of the other and within the context of a deeper field of connectedness. Buber writes,

> When I confront a human being as my 'Thou' and speak the basic word 'I–Thou' to him, then he is no thing among things nor does he consist of things. He is no longer 'He' or 'She', limited by other 'Hes' and 'Shes', a dot in the world grid of space and time, nor a condition that can be experienced and described, a loose bundle of named qualities. Persons now appear by entering into relation to other whole persons. (ibid., p. 15)

For Buber an I–Thou way of relating is a sacred process.

Assuming that we are embedded within a deeper field not only of sacred connectedness but also of the potentially desensitizing effects of personal, collective, and cultural assumptions, how can we, as clinicians, be truly present to our fellow humans? How can we as clinicians, caregivers, and educators come into an 'I–Thou' relationship with the people we care for and work with? Perhaps the first and necessary step is to engage in a process of resensitization.

The contribution of Buddhist psychology: Within a Buddhist worldview everything and everybody is ultimately interconnected, co-dependently arising and disappearing in a meaningful way. The view that we are autonomous individuals who can treat others as separate is seen as a misconception, a distortion of consciousness that leads to suffering for everyone involved. From a Buddhist perspective, therefore, the more we can be aware of our interconnectedness and live from that consciousness, the more peace and freedom we can have, experienced as kindness, generosity, and compassion.

Through the practice of Mindfulness Meditation we learn to attend to physical sensations and emotions, closely noticing as they arise, dissolve, and catalyse other feelings. We also learn to track when and how emotions trigger other reactions. In this way we come to see how all the processes of the mind are part of a larger interconnected process of perception. As we persist in our practice we may come to experience and see how our individual awareness is interconnected with other wider and deeper fields of consciousness. In this philosophy we ultimately do not exist in separateness and the fate of the individual affects others and the world at large. Learning to witness this process through mindful self-awareness can allow us to experience increased inner spaciousness and peace, and provide a possibility of living in balance within the bigger community of beings. Buddhist philosophy is not unique in having this perspective. Many of the mystical paths of the world's great religious traditions share the view of the interconnectedness of all beings and the meaning that needs to be found to find freedom. However, the Buddhist tradition does make available a number of meditative practices (such as those discussed above) that can be extremely useful in a contemporary clinical setting.

Exquisite Empathy: the practice of self-awareness in the present moment

Clinician self-awareness makes the practice of Exquisite Empathy in the moment possible. The practice of Exquisite Empathy involves focussed awareness, mindful self-awareness and dual-awareness in practice. It may be helpful to reflect on the different aspects of Exquisite Empathy as described by Harrison (2009) in more detail.

Highly present: Through Mindfulness Meditation we learn to hold focused attention in the present moment; noticing physical sensations, emotions, thoughts, and the environment we encounter, and to do so without being self-critical, judgemental, distracted, or impatient. Being mindfully present to physical and mental perception in this way grounds us in the present moment and in a heightened quality of presence. The relationship with our clients will then be qualitatively different because of this degree of presence.

Sensitively attuned: When the clinician has acquired self-knowledge, and through dual-awareness is mindful of both her- or himself and the client in a highly present and empathic way, then the clinician is able to attune to that particular client with great sensitivity. When sensitive attunement is practised within a cosmology of the interconnectedness and meaningfulness of life, we may notice how our lives are not separate from each other but instead are part of a much broader *gestalt*. This, in turn, may infuse the relationship with compassion and heighten the sensitivity of our attunement to the other.

Well-boundaried: Being 'well-boundaried' does not only mean holding the necessary legal and ethical boundaries. In a broader sense it also means knowing the limits of what one can and cannot do. The Serenity Prayer used by Alcoholics Anonymous says, 'May God grant me the serenity to accept the things I cannot change, the courage to change the things I can, and the wisdom to know the difference.' Making an accurate assessment of the clinical situation and accepting the limits of our clinical competence helps to create a safe container for the interaction, in which client and clinician can feel relaxed and open towards each other. Besides the obvious professional boundaries, clinicians also need to be aware of their internal limits and reserves, of what they can or cannot give. Sometimes the most compassionate thing to do is referral to someone else who can provide what is needed. 'Well-boundaried' might also mean awareness of transference feelings of the client towards the therapist as it rises in the moment of their meeting.

Heartfelt: Self-awareness also leads to an awareness of the state of our hearts. Most of us have habitually a shield of protection around our emotional core. Mindful self-awareness affords us a degree of emotional protection. Through the practice of mindful self-awareness we can learn to allow our shields to become more porous, our self-protection to be less rigid. While we are still protected when it is necessary, warmth can infuse the interpersonal dynamic allowing for the practice of Exquisite Empathy, and an 'I–Thou' relationship with the other person.

What does Exquisite Empathy look like at the bedside?

Dr X is an internist who is seen in clinical supervision. One day he talks about the case of Jodie, a 42-year-old woman, who was known to have carcinomatosis peritonei from a primary carcinoma of the cecum. Widowed five years earlier when her husband died of a malignant melanoma, she had two children and worked as a journalist. She had been brought up Roman Catholic but was no longer practising. When the doctor and nurse visited her at her home, they found a gaunt and frightened woman who complained of severe abdominal pain, nausea, and vomiting. Her family doctor had referred her to the palliative care unit for symptom management and emotional support while nearing the end of her life. Following admission even though physical condition stabilized, she became extremely emotionally distressed. 'This is the last straw,' she said, 'I feel utterly degraded . . . do you call this "dying with dignity"?'

Over the next few days Jodie remained greatly distressed and seemed inconsolable despite constant attention from her family and the ward staff. When Dr X sat down at her bedside, she told him, 'Doctor, what are you going to do to help me . . . I am in agony . . . even the stronger pain killers you gave me made no difference . . . I feel I am going crazy . . . nothing helps . . . I don't want to die . . . What have I done to deserve this? . . . promise me you won't let me die . . . Promise.'

During discussion with Dr X in clinical supervision, he remembered this as an extremely difficult situation for him. As we reflected on the situation, we realized that he could have reacted to Jodie in one of two ways. He could have avoided being with her by referring her to another physician or to other members of the interdisciplinary team (a *flight* reaction). Alternatively, he could have medicated Jodie to the point where she, and he, were out of pain (the *fight* reaction). In fact, he had done neither of these. He remembers feeling overwhelmed, numbed, and slightly dissociated (a *freeze* reaction), but it was at this point that his training in self-awareness proved to be immensely helpful.

Through *self-knowledge* he was able to recognize that he was extremely stressed and that he needed to step back, which he did by saying that, while he could sense her great distress, he was going to think about what else he could do to help her, and that he would come back to see her later that day. As he reflected on this situation he became aware that it always had been very hard for him to treat women who were the same age as his mother when she had died, and that the urge to save such women was extreme. His training in *self-empathy* allowed him to feel compassionate towards himself as he recognized the counter-transference in his feelings towards Jodie. This allowed him to feel more gentleness towards himself concerning his inability to help Jodie.

When reflecting on the contribution of his 12 years of training in Mindfulness Meditation, he could see how this made it a bit easier for him to stay present and emotionally open in a difficult situation without becoming detached, closed down, or self-critical. While sitting with Jodie in her despair, through *dual-awareness* he was able to distinguish her panic from his own distress and to identify his need to find a way of responding that would both offer her some reassurance and allow him to step back for now.

Dr X's spiritual understanding and the *contemplative awareness* this provided him with helped him to see that as humans we are not meaningless specks and that our lives are interconnected in mysterious ways we do not and perhaps cannot understand. It situated what was happening clinically in a bigger and deeper context. This allowed him to appreciate Jodie for who she was and to let her go to her journey as she entered uncharted territory and total uncertainty.

Dr X returned to Jodie's bedside and was part of her care in her final days. The capacities of self-awareness he had developed helped him to sit and be present with her in her suffering, without dissociating, feeling overwhelmed, or over-reacting. Even though Dr X was painfully aware of the limits of what he could do to help Jodie, she and her family commented on how valuable his support was. He remembers sitting with Jodie late one afternoon, holding her hand and breathing with her. He experienced a moment of peace, and it seemed that . . . Jodie did too.

In finishing, our hope and intention for this chapter is that it might help clinicians to engage empathically in more human, sensitive, and effective 'I–Thou' relationships, and that it might contribute to greater well-being, especially for those who are vulnerable.

References

Barrett-Leonard, G.T. (1997). Recovery of empathy: Toward self and others. In A.C. Bohart and L.S. Greenberg (eds), *Empathy Reconsidered: New Directions in Psychotherapy*. Washington DC: American Psychological Association.

Bloom, P. (2000). *Buddhist Acts of Compassion*. Berkeley, California: Conari Press, 157–63.

Buber, M. (1970). *I and Thou*, trans. Walter Kaufmann. New York: Charles Scribner's Sons.

Chodron, P. (2006). *Getting Unstuck*. Audiobook/CD: track 3. Boulder, CO: Sounds True Inc.

Figley, C.R. (ed.) (1995). *Compassion Fatigue: Coping with Secondary Traumatic Stress Disorder in Those who Treat the Traumatized*. New York: Brunner/Mazel.

Garfield, C., Spring, C., and Ober, D. (1995). *Sometimes My Heart Goes Numb: Caring in a Time of AIDS*. San Francisco: Jossey-Bass.

Harrison, R.L. and Westwood, M.J. (2009). Preventing vicarious traumatization of mental health therapists: Identifying protective practices. *Psychotherapy: Theory, Research, Practice, Training*, **46**(2), 203–19.

Hayes, J.A. (2004). Therapist know thyself: Recent research on countertransference. *Psychotherapy Bulletin*, **39**, 6–12.

Hojat, M., Gonnella, J.S., Nasca, T.J., Mangione, S., Vergare, M., and Magee, M. (2002). Physician empathy: Definition, components, measurement, and relationship to gender and specialty. *American Journal of Psychiatry*, **159**(9), 1563–69.

Kabat-Zinn, J. (2003). Mindfulness-based interventions in context: Past, present, and future. *Clinical Psychology Science Proceedings*, **10**(2), 144–55.

Kearney, M.K., Weininger, R.B., Vachon, M.L.S., Harrison, R.L., and Mount, B.M. (2009). Self-care of physicians caring for patients at the end of life. *Journal of the American Medical Association*, **301**(11), 1155–64.

Kornfield, J. (2008). *The Wise Heart: A Guide to the Universal Teachings of Buddhist Psychology*. New York: Bantam Books.

Maslach, C. and Leiter, M.P. (2008). Early predictors of job burnout and engagement. *Journal of Applied Psychology*, **93**(3), 498–512.

Maslach, C., Schaufeli, W.B., and Leiter, M.P. (2001). Job burnout. *Annual Review of Psychology*, **52**, 397–422.

Rothchild, B. (2000). *The Body Remembers: The Psychophysiology of Trauma and Trauma Treatment*. New York: W.W. Norton & Co.

Salzburg, S. (2008). *The Kindness Handbook: A Practical Companion*. Boulder, CO: Sounds True Inc.

Vachon, M.L.S. (2010). Oncology staff stress and related interventions. In J.C. Holland, W.S. Breitbart, and P.B. Jacobsen (eds), *Psycho-Oncology*, 2nd edn. New York: Oxford University Press, 2111–43.

Wallace, B.A. (2006). *The Attention Revolution: Unlocking the Power of the Focused Mind*. Somerville, MA: Wisdom Publications Inc.

Wright, B. (2004).Compassion fatigue: How to avoid it. *Palliative Medicine*, **18**(1), 4–5.

Chapter 5

Working and living with cancer, death, and dying: a personal reflection

Yvonne Yi Wood Mak

Introduction

I entered into palliative care thinking I could make a difference for the dying. Little did I know that in my giving, I have gained much more, as my patients have taught me invaluable lessons of life and how to be human. Palliative care is not confined to the clinical context but can be applied in our daily living. Its holistic approach can mould our attitudes and refine us into better caregivers and better persons, so palliative care is not just a profession but a way of life.

The constant exposure to death and dying can be emotionally threatening and over-whelming with negative feelings such as helplessness, guilt, and failure. Witnessing the suffering of others as well as experiencing our own empathic suffering can also be demoralizing. How do we care for the self when our work reminds us daily of such anguish, the fragility and brevity of life with its insecurities and uncertainties? How can we transform stress and suffering into strength and satisfaction?

We could deny this reality and concentrate on what we do well—communicating and comforting, managing symptoms, providing personal care, mobilizing resources, performing the last office, saying our prayers, and pretending that all is then settled. This seems professional and non-threatening as we do not need to expose our emotions. We can focus on the 'doing' part but we are not human 'doings', we are human 'beings'. We also need to learn how to 'be'.

Attending to our being is a way of self-care. This process of reflection and experiential learning not only promotes professional self-development by refining our tenor of care, but it also enhances self-awareness. It enables us to reflect and construct meaning in the midst of stress and struggles, reframe our attitudes and values, and redefine the self, thus promoting personal growth. If we allow ourselves to go through this thought-provoking and soul-searching exercise, reflective practice can transcend our stresses to build strengths with a positive outlook towards life and death, and our vulnerabilities can be used as healing tools to mould us into wounded healers.

The real challenge comes when our loved ones or we ourselves are faced with life-threatening illness. Yet, having practised palliative care, I was somehow equipped when my relatives and then I were struck down by cancer. I will share my personal journey as a physician, a relative, and a cancer patient, demonstrating how reflective practice has enabled me to (i) learn how to live as I care for the dying, (ii) care for others and self during stressful times, and (iii) use my wounds and vulnerabilities as healing tools to become a wounded healer. The art of palliative care can promote authentic living, and similarly personal lived experiences can enrich our art of care.

My professional journey: from stress to strength

In their vulnerability, they showed me courage to search for soul and meaning . . .
In their suffering, they taught me compassion to stand by and walk with them . . .
In their dying, they searched for serenity, for someone to hold and heal them . . .
As I listened, they became my greatest teachers on the meaning of life . . .
And in my search for knowledge they taught me wisdom—the meaning of being human . . .

(Mak, 2001, p. iii)

As I stepped into Bradbury Hospice, Hong Kong, for my first day of work, I felt confident in pain and symptom control. In my naivete, I thought that was what palliative medicine was all about. As I was waiting for the ward round, I started reading the patients' case notes. by the third one, I was in tears. The case histories were sad but were recorded with much depth and compassion. I soon realized I knew little about psychosocial care.

Over the years, I have come to appreciate the beauty of holistic care. I have chosen several stories to illustrate the patients' suffering and the caregivers' stress, and yet these encounters became useful experiential exercises for professional self-development.

It is okay to cry

I encountered a patient with pancreatic cancer and intractable neuropathic pain. The situation worsened when she suddenly developed cord compression and paraplegia. She felt useless and a sense of burden, and described her remaining existence as a bird in a cage. As she expressed a desire for death, it brought tears to my eyes. I could feel her pain and helplessness, but also my own sense of helplessness, for having failed her. A nurse comforted me: 'It's okay to cry. The patient feels you care and that you understand her pain. It shows you are human . . . ' I felt embarrassed but it was comforting to have been given the permission to cry . . . It prompted me to be more aware of my own feelings, fears, and failures, the need to address my emotions as well as those of my patients, and the need for team support.

Little acts of kindness

An elderly lady with maxillary cancer was transferred from an acute ward. She had previously tried to strangle herself with her nasogastric feeding tube. I have a vivid memory of our first encounter. Her face was so mummified with dressings that there was hardly a face to be seen. She had an Entriflex and her tracheostomy was covered with sputum. The referral stated she was deaf and blind but she could actually hear when we talked slowly and loudly, and she could see when the lighting was adequate.

She had facial pain, wound infection, sputum retention, and a pressure sore. The nurse and I examined her facial wound together, expecting to find a huge fungating wound. However, after removing the dressings, the facial disfigurement was not as bad as we had anticipated. The nurse refashioned the dressing so that it looked more presentable. The tender loving care and our acknowledgment of her distress comforted her and uplifted her sense of dignity and self-respect. We took time to listen to her and reassured her of our care.

I left her room thinking, 'If I had no face, no hearing, no vision, and no voice but instead a tracheostomy, an Entriflex, and were bed bound with a bed sore, I would want to die too . . . ' Her distress was unbearable but on the following morning she told me, 'I'm very happy!' With good symptom control, excellent nursing care, patience, and attention to detail, she no longer desired death.

Her remaining days were meaningful as her relatives showed her their last acts of love and care, and she had the opportunity to express her last words. I was encouraged to see how palliative care could make such a difference in such a short space of time. However hopeless the situation may seem, we can make a difference.

Holding and not abandoning

Young, beautiful Amy was dying. Her mother arrived from China and was heartbroken, seeing her daughter so emaciated. She stayed with Amy day and night, massaging and applying a hot pad to wherever there was pain.

One morning, when I was doing my ward round, I found Amy's bedside curtain half-drawn. As I peeped through, I saw Mum lying in bed with Amy, stroking her hair. It was like a mother stroking her newborn and the baby was all cuddled up in the comfort of the mother's embrace. The connectedness was so strong and they seemed inseparable despite such intense grief.

Mum was weeping quietly and her eyes were all swollen. As I could not speak her dialect, all I could do was to hold her hand, and I placed my other hand over her shoulder. She held on tightly to my hand and would not let go. The room was dead silent but we were communicating—through our tears. I sensed she needed my support, but more so, she wanted me to save Amy. She was not ready to let go of her, just as she would not let go of my hand. I stood there for ten minutes. Then a nurse walked in and, noticing that we were both crying, handed us some tissues. I asked the nurse to tell Mum that Amy was comfortable and that the team would continue to care for her. I did not know what comforting words to say . . . Finally I got hold of Amy's hand and placed it into Mum's hand so that she would finally let go of mine . . .

Mum's love was unconditional; she was fully connected and non-abandoning. She portrayed the essence of palliative care—to affirm life, to be present, to be willing to suffer with the sufferer, to stay connected without abandoning. Embracing death can be so painful and yet it can also be so beautiful.

Meaning of suffering

A gentleman with metastatic cancer had previously tried to commit suicide on the oncology ward as his pain was unbearable. However, he had promised his daughter he would give life one more chance for another month and he seemed at peace when he arrived on our ward. Within days, his physical symptoms were controlled. However, he had unresolved grief from the deaths of two close relatives. He declined psychological counselling, so this was respected.

Over the next few weeks his mobility deteriorated. Despite being symptom-free, he requested euthanasia. On further exploration, he anticipated he would die in overwhelming distress with intractable symptoms. He felt helpless over his disease with a sense of lack of control. He feared increasing dependency and his remaining days seemed hopeless and meaningless. He had masked depression but the depressive symptoms became apparent during his request. We could sense his anguish which also extended to the team. Antidepressants were commenced and we continued our support and counselling.

One week later he made another euthanasia request. He declined going over issues such as his fears and unresolved grief. His extreme anguish together with my own sense of helplessness and empathic suffering nearly pushed me to want to do 'something.' He said,

> There's nothing left for me to do now . . . A month's up and God's abandoned me! I'm still suffering! All the patients have died comfortably but that won't happen in my case. No doctor and nobody can help me . . . Give me an injection and let me die now! If you can't do that, make me physically stronger so that I can do it myself!

After further negotiation, he consented to be temporarily sedated. He agreed to be woken up for his antidepressant medication and for some food and drink. Daytime sedation was then gradually reduced with his agreement and this allowed further counselling. A week before he died, his mood was more stable. He thanked the team and then asked for me. As soon as I arrived, he held my hands tightly, telling me that he did not want to die at all, and he thanked me for not abandoning him during his times of emotional anguish. He was so genuine and appreciative that it brought tears to my eyes. I thanked him for his honesty and for sharing his vulnerabilities with us.

I was relieved I did not heed his request. I pondered, 'What is his suffering?' His euthanasia request signified the intensity of suffering. The meaning of suffering is individualized and multi-dimensional. It is not solely about physical pain and dependency but hidden fears and the psycho-spiritual impact of the disease progression on his whole being, leading to disintegration of personhood and the existential distress of feeling hopeless, meaningless, a burden, and worthless, coupled with depression, unfulfilled wishes, past life experiences, and unresolved grief.

The hospice provided a safe place to contain his suffering. We acknowledged his suffering and he felt understood. We provided counselling according to his pace. In times of extreme anguish, temporary sedation was used without the intention to hasten death. Despite his suffering and the empathic suffering that we also felt, we did not abandon him. Our helplessness could have pushed us into thinking that euthanasia was a compassionate way of relieving suffering, but his words of gratitude confirmed the contrary.

This gentleman placed a passion in my heart to explore the meaning behind the patient's desire for death. If it were not for him, I would have taken these requests at face value; I would not have paid attention to the meaning of suffering; I would not have transcended my own suffering to find an interest in existential care. 'Thank you for being my greatest teacher!'

Lessons learned: care for self and others

Having witnessed how my patients embrace death, I view life from a completely different perspective that is more genuine and authentic. They have been my inspiration on the meaning of suffering and also the meaning of life. They have taught me courage to face one's wounds and vulnerabilities, to forget and forgive, to grasp the opportunity to say 'Sorry' and 'Thank you'. They have shown me the importance of relationships and the need to stay connected. They have shown me the wisdom of when to hold on and let go in order to have inner peace. They have shown me how personal growth is possible despite physical disintegration and how suffering can be transcended to reach healing. They have taught me how to be resilient—to be flexible, to accept the reality but stay hopeful, to live in the moment, and appreciate the little things. Even their anger, rigid personalities, and regrets have been meaningful lessons.

My colleagues have nurtured me, showing me how to care with patience, kindness, and gentleness, to listen more than we should speak, without being judgemental but to accept and respect the person as he or she is. They have shown me many virtues of a caregiver—presence, honesty, trustworthiness, genuineness, empathy, compassion, and non-abandonment.

The hospice and my colleagues provided a secure holding environment for personal growth. Self-awareness is the key to self-care. In order to transcend my work-related stress and struggles, this safe space allowed me to address my suffering, examine my actions and reactions, and reflect on my thoughts and feelings at my own pace. I could re-evaluate my attitudes and assumptions, reframe my tenor of care, and cultivate virtues needed for the care of the dying. This process of deep self-exploration enabled me to construct meaning and also find healing. Without it, the accumulation of much emotional burden would have caused burnout and compassion fatigue.

Many colleagues might have experienced other life events at work or in their personal lives, not necessarily life-threatening but significant enough to cause possible burnout or compassion fatigue. Thus the awareness of symptoms of burnout and staff support are essential in sustaining the well-being of the whole team. While one is overwhelmed, work is redistributed to lessen the burden. When one is burnt out, there must be time out. While one is wounded, others need to step in to facilitate healing, just as while one-winged angels cannot fly, if they hold hands, together they can.

Conducting formal reflection days and self-care workshops, debriefing, and reflective practice sessions for the multi-disciplinary team are important for self-care and professional self-development. The caregiver's work and life experiences are invariably intertwined—what one has learned at work could be applied in personal life and vice versa. Every colleague is unique with his or her individualized set of gifts and inner resources gained from personal or professional experiences that could help to support and revitalize other members of the team. A trusting relationship and non-judgemental attitude are vital so that a safe space is created for personal sharing. Seniors need the sensitivity and awareness that their presence could be threatening for the frontline and support groups might be better conducted in their absence.

Informal mutual support is just as relevant as formal sessions. Those sharing the same religion would find comfort and encouragement from one another. The creative aspects of each individual staff member can bring cohesiveness and cultivate a harmonious environment. Activities such as weekend retreats, hiking, enjoying home-made bread, cakes, savouries, and sweets, exchanging recipes, hosting cooking lessons, beadwork, knitting, crochet, and other arts and crafts are good diversion therapies. They create a sense of wholeness for the team and also an opportunity to know the person beyond the professional.

My personal journey as a relative: from suffering to surrendering

What a week! Dad has had so many tests . . . As I was walking behind Mum and Dad, for the first time, it suddenly hit me how old they actually are. They were walking slowly and suddenly they seemed so much frailer . . . I am no longer dependent on them, something which I've taken for granted. There seems a sudden role reversal—they are now dependent and I've become a carer . . . (My diary, August 2002)

In 2002, my father was diagnosed with cancer. It never crossed my mind that cancer could knock at my family's door. I began to experience the suffering of a relative. It was physically and emotionally draining and I felt unconfident in how to care even though I knew how to. I also felt fears of anticipatory loss. I had never realized the dilemmas and burdens of decision-making as I now had to, bearing the personal consequences if those decisions turned out to be wrong. The empathic suffering of witnessing my father going through his chemotherapy and radiotherapy—the cachexia, anorexia, vomiting, and tiredness—was heartbreaking (Mak 2005). I thought he would miss his hair, so I had my long hair cut short.

I asked myself, 'Do I practise what I preach?' I applied the art of palliative care on my family, for example, how to communicate effectively and sensitively, how to be present, stay connected without abandoning, respect and be non-judgemental, empathize and be compassionate; and how to be flexible and appreciative, taking a day at a time.

I took time to reflect by recording my experience as a relative. Diary-keeping helped to externalize my grief. I became aware of my behaviour, emotions, grief, and how my relatives were reacting. 'What am I doing?' 'Why am I doing this?' 'How am I feeling?' 'Why are others saying things and behaving the way they are?' Writing helped me to make sense of and surrender to my circumstances. I have included several raw excerpts from my diary to illustrate the flow of fleeting thoughts, reflections, and meaning-making, reframing and moving forward. These writings may not have correct grammar or separate paragraphs but they were expressed spontaneously from my pen without my mind processing what my hand was writing.

A relative's stress

'Everyone is so different and I'm constantly switching from one mode to another . . . My job has been advocating for Dad's needs and comforting (sometimes confronting) Mum, letting her be more aware of his needs, and then go back to Dad and tell him about Mum's perspective, and suggest they should both take it easy. It's been hard and so tiring—being a facilitator, a daughter, having to soak up everyone's emotions and control my own, witnessing Dad going through his treatments, lack of sleep . . . but Sis is great; she is so practical . . . ' (My diary, October 2002).

Insecurity or *serenity*

'Where am I going? I'm drifting and waiting for God to show me the way. I'm like a kite on a string, getting blown around by the wind, not having any direction in my own way. Is this insecurity or serenity—having the freedom to fly, held by the string of God, but the uncertainty of not knowing where I would end up?' (My diary, December 2002).

Year of suffering, surrendering, and surrounding

I've learned to surrender—to let go of things on Earth, for they are being taken away from me . . . let go of my loved ones—for they are slowly fading away . . . let go of my chores— as what seems worthwhile today would be futile tomorrow . . . I live a day at a time . . . I've learned to love—just to hold you a little closer, a little tighter, and a little longer . . . I have learned to trust God in the midst of my burdens . . . I have learned to count my blessings and have the courage to make breakthroughs which I wouldn't have tried otherwise. I have witnessed little miracles through the power of prayer, so I pray even for the tiniest things, hoping God would hear and hold me . . . So it has been a year of suffering, sur-rendering, and surrounding. In my letting go of what I thought I needed, instead I have become surrounded by a precious kind of love, and I have found healing and peace at the end of the tunnel. That's my lesson from the Chinese Year of the Horse. As I look forward to the Year of the Sheep, I pray there will be a shepherd leading the way. A horse can end up running wild; the sheep is stupid but has a shepherd . . . Admire and be inspired by the beauty of music . . . I love the feeling of music—it gives me wings to fly and the power to dream . . . Refine the heart with virtues . . . Believe in the power of the dream and the power of prayer . . . (My diary, February 2003).

Lessons learned

I learned new lessons observing how my father had coped with his cancer. He was my great mentor. He accepted the reality and said, 'I know I have to suffer but it is nothing compared to what Jesus had to suffer on the cross.' He did not focus on his own suffering but the suffering of others. He persevered during his treatment; he never moaned nor got angry. He had an inner calm. He was appreciative and counted his blessings. When his treatments were over, he said, 'I am not going to worry about whether or not those cancer cells will recur but I will treasure my days remaining.' Witnessing his relational connectedness with God through continual prayers, it seemed as if he had an eternal rechargeable battery to draw strength from.

I had many soul-searching questions. I could not understand why one had to suf-fer until I had personally experienced suffering as a relative. I concluded, 'Suffering is inevitable but not in vain, for where there is love, there will be suffering. I would rather have a world with suffering than a world without love.' I began to embrace death experientially rather than intellectually. I surrendered to the brevity of life, its insecurities and uncertainties. I learned to let go of my losses, parts of my old self, and situations that were preventing me from moving forward. I reset my roles and priorities. I cherished my moments with my loved ones. I re-evaluated my values, learning to trust beyond human understanding. Paradoxically, by embracing death, I began to experience an authentic way of living (Mak, 2005).

My personal journey as a cancer patient: from vulnerabilities to virtues

In September, 2003, I fell and fractured my sacrum. The fall was the beginning of a transition from being a physician who was accustomed to relieving the pain of her cancer patients, to a patient who was personally experiencing excruciating pain. The real challenge began when I developed breast cancer two months later, having to personally experience all the vulnerabilities and suffering as a patient. It was a very testing time but it was also a time to rest, reflect, re-pace, and reprioritize my life. I applied the lessons I had learned from palliative care and from my relatives. Overall, my cancer journey has enabled me to mature as a person and suffering has transformed me into a wounded healer. I have included excerpts from my diary, illustrating the ways I tried to stay resilient, appreciate the support I had, and also construct meaning out of my suffering (Mak, 2006).

My emotions

Although I had witnessed how cancer patients had coped with courage, a positive attitude, composure, and faith, it did not prevent me from experiencing all the psychological reactions of numbness, shock, fear, despair, and grief. It was important to acknowledge those natural emotions but at the same time to try to move forward.

> I felt numb, physically exhausted, and emotionally overwhelmed by fear and the thought of death. I was trembling . . . I took a sleeping pill but couldn't sleep. I got up the following morning and curled up into a ball on my bed. I thought, 'The body is so vulnerable; it has ended up with cells that have become out of control.' Outwardly I appeared calm but I knew my blood pressure was up, my heart pounding, my muscles tense, and my teeth chattering. Doom preoccupied my mind. I grieved and it was not about my own eventual mortality but what gave me most pain was the thought of separation. It felt as if everyone was dying and I was the one being left behind. A relative would only have to grieve for the loss of a loved one, but I would have to grieve for all the ones I love, a much heavier loss and pain. This brought tears to my eyes . . . I reached out for a book lying on my bedside table and the first thing I read was a Bible verse, 'I have plans for you . . . plans to prosper you and not to harm you, plans to give you a hope and a future.' This somehow spoke to me and brought me comfort. I said to myself, 'My cancer is not meant to harm me!' I opened another book and the same verse popped up! Wow! This was incredible! The following day, the verse appeared for the third time! This reassurance brought me tremendous calmness. 'I will live! I'll live!' (Adapted from Mak, 2006, pp. 24–5)

My Oasis

Whatever the circumstances, creating an oasis provided a sense of control and contentment. My oasis consisted of resources where I could continue to learn and at the same time 'enjoy' being ill.

> Since I will spend my next six months at home, I have created my own little oasis in my bedroom with a sea view, music, DVDs, photos, books, journals, aromatherapy, notepads, and computer. So my room is fully equipped. I imagine myself becoming a newborn baby with no hair and no immunity, having small and frequent feeds with everything cooked and sterilised. I will not have much autonomy but lots of sleep, educational toys and pampering when I am awake. Everybody will be babbling on the phone, trying to cheer me up, but they will have no idea what this baby is really up to! (Adapted from Mak, 2006, p. 46)

My holding environment

I defined my holding environment that would keep me safe and connected. This consisted of my family, colleagues, and church friends from both near and far, their support and prayers, communication with others through email and with the self through reflective writing, and my personal faith.

> I've never felt so supported by so many. The phone kept ringing; cards, chocolates, flowers and presents keep coming in. I was deeply touched . . . Many knew exactly what I needed without my asking. They did not need to be physically present but were empathic and would respond willingly in a second to my needs. What I appreciated most were e-mails, as I could read and reply to them at my own pace. Many friends and colleagues knew just the right words to say and the right time to send them . . . One wrote, 'I know that you are warmly wrapped in the secure blanket of everyone's love and I cannot think of a greater sanctuary.' Another wrote, 'While I won't insult your medical intelligence by saying that 'everything will be all right', the likelihood is that it will be. I see so many women at clinics now who are many years out from diagnosis and who remain in excellent health.' (Adapted from Mak, 2006, pp. 41–2)

Creative writing

Creative writing was an extremely therapeutic and useful resource during my cancer journey. My diary contained emails, quotes from books and films, conversations, and personal reflections.

> As I began recording my thoughts and feelings, the diary became a mirror of my inner self . . . My diary was a 'great listener' as it never made any insensitive comments nor ever got offended. It never interrupted me but was always ready to receive whatever I had to tell. If I have been too harsh, I could take them back and they were never remembered. Later on, when I reflected on what I had scribbled, I tried to make sense of my suffering and find meaning amidst my life of mess in a calm and constructive manner, so my writing has become a transcribed personal journey of struggles and sweet memories, existential quests and enlightenments, reflections and revelations. This process of recording, reading, and reflecting has provided a channel through which I could connect with my inner self, gain self-awareness, and reframe my mind . . . (Adapted from Mak, 2006, p. 10)

My vulnerabilities

My vulnerabilities humbled me and made me more aware of the fragility of other cancer patients. This awareness is difficult to teach but has to be experienced.

> Many say I look fine . . . but the world cannot see the 'me' that is inside this superficial body shell. I am living in pretence. Outwardly, this 'shell' wears make-up, nail varnish, a wig, fancy clothes, and a smile, but inwardly, no one sees that battered battery, the head without my wig, the disfigured and discoloured body underneath my clothes. No one knows about my hot flushes and insomnia during the night, my joint pain when I wake up and my wobbly quadriceps when I walk. They are unaware of the emotional unrest underneath my apparent calmness, the vulnerabilities behind my every smile, and fears when my faith feels so distant. I don't feel like a woman as the chemo has induced a temporary menopausal state. Only those who understand the inner world of a patient would be sensitive enough to ask, 'Do you feel as well as you look?' (Adapted from Mak, 2006, p. 114)

What am I?

Having experienced suffering personally as a physician, relative, and patient, my vulnerabilities have transformed me into a wounded healer. Paradoxically, wounds can become instruments of healing, enabling us to understand the wounds of others so that they may find healing through us.

> As I stepped into Bradbury after bringing closure to my cancer journey, I was perplexed and anxious but also excited. I asked myself, not 'Who am I?' but 'What am I?' 'Am I a physician, a researcher, a relative or a patient?' Then a small inner voice whispered, 'You are a person!' It seems I have acquired an extra medical qualification and I can literally say to my cancer patients, 'I know exactly what you mean and I know exactly how you feel.' (Adapted from Mak, 2006, p. 118)

We are effective healers when we have processed our wounds and vulnerabilities. Personal suffering is a humbling experience. Our vulnerabilities can increase our awareness, sensitivity, and openness to the suffering of others, which make us more compassionate to share deeper levels of inner pain. We are more able to accept uncertainty, take risks with our patients, thus providing a deeper connection and greater intimacy (Boston and Mount, 2006).

Lessons of life

My cancer experience was an awakening. It refined me and redefined the person I wanted to be. Adversities in life can be turned into invaluable lessons of life if we maintain a positive attitude to our suffering.

> Slow down and be still . . . Be disciplined and learn to listen . . . Attend to the body, mind and soul . . . Do not demand but be specific with your needs . . . As no one can ever fully understand another, change yourself and not others . . . Do not victimise yourself but let go of self-pity . . . Don't hold onto anger or it will hold onto you . . . If you forgive, your burdens will fly away . . . Do not dwell on negative thoughts, feelings and situations; acknowledge them and then let them go . . . Feelings are unreliable and can distort reality . . . Stay positive and count your blessings in disguise . . . Let go of your old self and frustrations . . . Learn to

live with it or live without . . . Live in the present moment of the here and now . . . Create your own oasis . . . Do not rely on your own strength but have a jump lead connected to heaven . . . Bank all your precious memories . . . Focus on others rather than on yourself . . . You have not suffered in vain. We do not live to suffer but we suffer in order to learn to live . . . Comfort and edify others . . . Cancer is not a death sentence but an opportunity to be a new self and have a new life. (Adapted from Mak, 2006, p. 161)

These principles on authentic living sound almost too ideal and unrealistic, as my patients are like a thorn in my heart that reminds me daily of life's fragility and uncertainties, and the inevitability of death. I have to admit that my fears and vulnerabilities continue to overwhelm me from time to time, as I anticipate my own cancer recurrence or the death of my loved ones. I can only try my best and learn to appreciate my blessings, the little things, and the here and now.

Conclusion

These patient stories and excerpts from my diary have shown that suffering can be transcended into healing when we allow ourselves to connect with our wounds and vulnerabilities and to use them as tools to re-evaluate our values, attitudes, and assumptions, and construct meaning out of every seemingly dreadful experience. This not only refines our tenor of care for our patients but it also promotes self-care and enables us to live more authentic lives. While I would not wish it on anyone to have to go through my experience in order to become wounded healers, a less threatening method is to attend to spiritual care and make use of non-medical literary sources such as art, literature, films, and music to understand more about the human experience, illness, dying, and bereavement. Even the ordinary everydayness has something to teach us if we enhance our awareness and are more mindful. It is important to keep a positive attitude regardless of our circumstances and believe in the transcendent power of suffering in bringing healing for the self and others.

References

Boston, P.H. and Mount, B.M. (2006). The caregiver's perspective on existential and spiritual distress in palliative care. *Journal of Pain and Symptom Management*, **32**, 13–26.

Mak, Y.Y.W. (2001). Meaning of desire for euthanasia in Chinese advanced cancer patients: a hermeneutic study. MSc in Palliative Medicine, University College of Wales.

Mak, Y.Y.W. (2005). A personal journey: The professional, relative, researcher and patient. In C. Chan and A. Chow (eds), *Death, Dying and Bereavement*. Hong Kong: Hong Kong University Press, 31–64.

Mak, Y.Y.W. (2006). *Dr. Hannah: A Mother's Diary—Chronicle of Life and Faith through Cancer*. Hong Kong: Swindon Books.

Chapter 6

Jumping the fence: the impact of a life-threatening illness in the workplace

Ann Saville and Rosemary Feeley

Not welcome
Hijack; kidnap all that is me,
Leave me bare, take all I am
Shuffle, spin, turn
And return me to my ground,
Shake, uncertain, unfamiliar
Not welcome.
(Excerpt from the poem 'A Letter to Cancer', Ann Saville, May 2007)

Introduction

In this chapter we have adopted a narrative approach to describe the impact of a life-threatening illness in a palliative care workplace when, as social work colleagues, one of us was diagnosed and treated for cancer and the other thrust into a supportive role. We will explore some of the lessons and issues associated with this experience and discuss the implications for both management and staff when faced with such a challenge.

Gunaratam and Oliviere (2009), have emphasized the importance of narrative-based evidence and the value of storytelling in providing insight and clarity to the confusion experienced during a serious illness. Since the narrative approach has always been our preferred way of working as social workers in palliative care, we decided that this would be the best way to explore the topic of caregiver stress and staff support. We will show that a narrative approach has as much value in documenting a workplace crisis as it does in highlighting the issues that are central to patient and family care. As Arthur Frank (1995) suggests in *The Wounded Storyteller*, 'illness is a call for stories.'

When developing a best-practice support model in the workplace for people with a life-threatening illness and employed carers, Bottomley and Tehan (2005) used the narrative approach to provide insights into what kind of support would be of most benefit. They found that the narrative approach not only helped to reveal both the unique and shared experiences of work, illness, and support but also guided them in developing a framework for a best-practice model.

Ann's story

When Rosemary and I first began working together in a community-based palliative care programme we were both mature and experienced social workers and felt well prepared for a role that involved constant exposure to death, dying, and bereavement. The palliative care programme was about to change its model of practice, moving from a predominantly medical model to one which placed a greater emphasis on psychosocial and holistic care. However, in December 2006 we were confronted with a crisis when I was diagnosed with a life-threatening illness, breast cancer. There was now a new story to be told. We were no longer observers and narrators, but the main characters in this confronting experience. In an article published in *Illness, Crisis and Loss* (2010) I describe the following reactions:

> I was overwhelmed with disbelief at the possibilities. I was numb, empty, and speechless. I felt that if I spoke about it, it would become more real. I silenced myself because it was Christmas and I had to perform my role and duties. I couldn't acknowledge the possibility that I might have cancer. I was to visit the experience of being silenced so often over the next twelve months as I confronted my fears and disbeliefs, and endured the effects of treatments that would leave me unable to communicate. It was about to be my family's first Christmas without my father who had passed away just two months earlier. We were still raw with grief from his death and now this? (Saville, 2010)

My experience had given us a unique opportunity to reflect on the issues of caregiver stress and staff support when working within a palliative care setting. Whether it was in our work with clients, or the work of supporting each other as colleagues and members of a caring team, we were able to learn about the things that provide support and strength when a colleague is forced to 'jump the fence' into an illness experience (Saville, 2010).

> And, so, I had 'jumped the fence', as one of my clients so richly reminded me. My employer had sent a letter to my clients saying that due to unexpected circumstances, I would not be able to continue working with them. Not long after this I bumped into one of my clients who gently berated me with the words, 'So you've abandoned us'. When I explained why I had taken leave she said lovingly and with great compassion, 'It's OK. You've just jumped the fence.' It was a quiet and flawless statement so exquisite in its authenticity and accuracy to my experience. It would lead me to investigate the use of metaphoric language that surrounds illness and disease. This experience of cancer has forced me to review all aspects of my life, both the personal and the professional: how I have lived as a person and how I wish to live it in the future, and how I have worked as a professional and will work in my practice from now on.

It was when my cancer diagnosis removed the security of distance and detachment that our professional and personal worlds collided. As I entered the world of the client, Rosemary entered the world of the caregiver. It was at that time that the notion of mirroring came to mind. To 'mirror' is defined in the *Oxford English Dictionary* as a verb, to 'show a reflection of' or to 'correspond to'. We felt that the experience of one of us as the colleague with the life-threatening illness, and the other as colleague in a support role, while both working in a palliative care setting, was at times a mirror image of the experiences of chaos, shock, and fear that were constantly reported by our clients.

The boundaries between the roles of the professional and the client, and 'who was who', were no longer clearly defined. Deep down there had been unspoken feelings of immortality, of being somehow untouchable or immune to the realities of life and death. Papadatou (2009) says that caregivers privatize their pain in silence and remain dissociated and estranged from themselves to protect themselves from knowing how they are being affected by the grief experiences of others. She also speaks of a 'death presence where we do not deny death, but only acknowledge its existence in the world of our clients—a world we visit briefly in a detached manner, for fear of contamination' (Papadatou, 2009, pp. 40–1). Youngson (2009) refers to the way that practitioners can retreat to a place of supposed emotional detachment. Papadatou (2009) reminds us that we are 'human and equal in the face of death' and are confronted and made painfully aware of our own mortality, our own losses. Halifax (2008) talks about the bonds of 'impermanence' when we are working with the dying that remind us that we are all linked by the inevitability of loss and grief, even if we are walking the road of the living. In the words of Emily Dickinson,

> Because I could not stop for death
> He kindly stopped for me
> The carriage held but just ourselves
> And immortality
> (Reeves, 1959, p. 65)

Rosemary's story

Both of us experienced a void, an amplified helplessness, a frozen state in our grief response. As I witnessed Ann's diagnosis I experienced a wide range of emotions including anger, blaming, and tearfulness. They were emotions and responses I had witnessed daily within the intimate sacred space of many of the homes of the families with whom I worked. The physical loss of my work colleague was reflected in the angst of my daily working life. I needed to make sense of this process through reflective practice and with professional supervision in order to be able to continue to be available to my clients whilst struggling with my personal distress. I wondered how I would be able to continue caring for others, while confronted daily with Ann's empty desk in the office that we shared without the shared compassion and conversations about how we were 'travelling' emotionally each day.

I experienced a silence in the office and in the corridors of the organization as I was fearful about expressing my emotions and felt the need to keep soldiering on in an environment of stoicism. Coupland and Raphael (2009) reflect on the concept of 'empathic muting' and the question of how workers keep it together in palliative care when one must suspend one's feelings to enable the caring to continue and avoid being seen as not coping.

At the same time as I was coping with Ann's absence I also lost my line manager who had moved from the organization. At times I felt like I was onboard a ship without a rudder. So began for me a constant search for some meaning amongst the chaos, an experience that Ann shared as she took leave from the workplace to commence a series of surgeries and treatments for her cancer. We both experienced overwhelming grief in that search for meaning amongst the onslaught of emotion. We felt that we were experiencing a kind of disenfranchized grief. Doka (1989) defines disenfranchized grief as the hidden sorrows associated with loss not visibly identifiable to the world.

As Ann started her treatment, I rushed off to an overseas hospice conference looking for answers. In a two-week period I searched for different ways in which hospice and palliative care could be offered. I wondered how I could 'bottle' the things I'd heard and seen so that the benefits would continue to affect my work in palliative care. I felt like a 'mad woman' coming back to work, high on adrenalin but still overwhelmed by the experience of Ann's situation. The experiences of visiting and learning about palliative care services in England, Scotland, and Ireland and their approaches to palliative care had brought some relief from the personal and professional pain I had been experiencing. But not long after returning, I realized it had been only a snapshot view, and also just how grief stricken I had been. It had been a search to try to 'fix' something that was viable and more concrete from an organizational perspective, but in reality I think I was trying to 'fix' myself. I recall being reminded of images of Venetian masks, masks that remind us that we are all different people living in different environments, and that we may at times hide behind these masks to protect us from our own personal and professional pain. It is only in a safe environment that we are able to freely express emotions. Cicely Saunders is cited in *The Tibetan Book of Living and Dying* (Rinpoche, 1992) as saying that 'the dying have shed their masks and superficial ties of everyday living and they are all the more open and sensitive because of this' (p. 211). In the workplace, many special people died during this time. I was confronted with the fact that I was working in an environment where one returns from leave to learn of the loss of many families. The reality is that one's case load only shrinks due to death. There seemed to be a merging of the accumulated stress and grief associated with the work of caring for patients and families together with my anguish about my dear friend and colleague.

It was a struggle to understand team culture at times. I wondered how to articulate a range of emotions and grief responses within the work environment and how to relate to the other colleagues with whom Ann had developed close collegial relationships. I felt the loss of Ann as a close colleague at a personal level but also as a skilled member of our team; and still further, I was aware of Ann's own losses as she faced the unknown.

I should add that despite the daily confrontations with death and suffering, working in palliative care has certainly enriched my life and enabled me to 'make meaning' in many difficult circumstances. Kauffman (1995) refers to meaning making as a way of enriching workers' personal lives and offering them new horizons.

The workplace

Papadatou (2009) explains how organizations develop a culture which regulates suffering within the organization, telling us how to act, fit in, and behave just as team dynamics can also mirror the dynamics experienced by families in the face of loss and separation. Within the workplace both of us had witnessed the team mirroring the experience of the personal chaos so often described by their clients.

Running parallel to the personal health crisis we have described was the organizational change from a bio-medical model of care to a more holistic model. We were also moving from a multi-disciplinary to an interdisciplinary way of practice. Ovretveit (1996) defines the multi-disciplinary teams as one where there is a variety of interprofessional working arrangements.

Organizational change and financial pressures on the healthcare system are creating new imperatives for interdisciplinary teamwork (Baldwin, 1994). Interdisciplinary teams require well-coordinated collaboration across all professions involved. It is argued that what is required is a culture of support and openness. Following the death of his wife, Charles-Edwards (2009) felt that the most crucial element in helping him through the bereavement within his workplace was the support he received from his line manager and his colleagues. Tehan (Bottomley and Tehan, 2005) adds that, if expressions of grief are considered a 'taboo' in the workplace, the worker with the life-threatening illness or their carer may feel discriminated against and even further stigmatized. Papadatou's (2009, p. 257) concept of the 'trans-disciplinary team' would therefore seem to be a more compassionate model for the workplace, since it is a team that 'evolves and goes through stages of development that allows for increasing degrees of openness'.

We were indeed fortunate that we had a leader who was able to acknowledge the personal grief that was being experienced and was aware of the needs for support for all members of our team. There was sensitivity to our needs while remaining focused on the bigger picture as a leader. On reflection we can now appreciate how hard this must have been for the senior management team who needed to keep the work of the organization going. The organization called on assistance from an external Employees Assistance Programme (EAP), a model which provides employees with grief support and stress management by trained counsellors whose services are engaged for a limited time. However, Bottomley (2009) warns that this approach may result in grief 'being quarantined' and kept apart from the workplace, as the grieving employee is relocated to a clinical setting while the work ideology is left unchallenged.

Charles-Edwards (2009) identifies the additional stress that may be experienced when a work culture changes due to mergers or changes in service delivery models, but also suggests that this stress can be reduced, depending on the quality of the working relationships, trust, honesty, and management style. In our case senior management took on the role of liaising directly with Ann, taking advice from her about how and when to update other staff members. According to Tehan (2005) a best-practice support model is one which adopts a person-centred approach and which provides managers with strategies to keep the employee at the centre of their decision-making while also carrying out their responsibilities to the organization as a whole.

Wolfelt (2005) stresses the need for workplace managers to create a culture of compassion, and this was to be our experience. Ann continued to be included in the team and the agency despite being unable to continue in her usual role. Generous offers to 'just come and shuffle papers' were made, if the need was felt. Ann received invitations to team events and continued to be seen as an integral part of the agency. Charles-Edwards (2009) explains that managers have a dual role. They need to attend to the needs of the business as well as those of the individual. They are required to combine task- and person-centered approaches so that the individual feels that the workplace is committed to them as a human being. Tehan (2005) also describes this need for humanity to co-exist with meeting the production needs in an atmosphere of mutuality. Management's support for Rosemary's request to have the Employees Assistance Program conduct a debriefing session was an indication of such an approach. The debriefing allowed all nursing and medical staff, volunteers, and members of the psychosocial/spiritual care team to explore their experience as a whole without fragmenting and privatizing their experience. Rosemary felt this gave permission for the sharing of tears, anger, and other emotions, although this was at times confrontational. Charles-Edwards (2009) suggests that managers need to be 'emotionally literate' in order to understand the behaviours that may be exhibited in the workplace in the light of a bereavement situation or some other critical event.

The following is an account of some of the ways in which we coped with the crisis of Ann's illness. We explore the use of metaphor, the practice of mindfulness, and the value of external supervision and support.

Life rafts and light houses: the power of metaphor

Since we shared a common professional background there was a shared understanding of language, theoretical perspectives, work ethics, codes of practice, and values that somehow created a 'life raft' to which we were able to cling as we worked together. Our office became a sanctuary in which we shared stories of our clients and their experiences of grief, sadness, and despair. We had daily opportunities for authentic sharing of the impact of the work and for mutual support which prevented or at least mitigated against compassion fatigue. Keidel (2002) defines compassion fatigue in palliative care as arising when hospice workers experience personal sources of pressure outside the hospice environment such as societal pressures, frustrations with healthcare systems, deficits of support or education, or troubled interpersonal relationships. It is also defined as the 'daily struggle to narrow the gap between the "real" and the "ideal" and to balance the level of intimacy associated with empathic involvement . . . the cumulative impact of dealing with many terminally ill patients at the same time . . . '

We reflected on the language we shared and the language of metaphor that became so important to us in coping with the crisis triggered by Ann's illness. Reisfield and Wilson (2004) note that metaphors can assist both physicians and patients as the language of metaphor provides a basis for the shared understanding of clinical reality in the therapeutic relationship. The shared metaphoric rapport can help in communicating the unshared experience. Penson et al. (2004) also point out the benefits for both the client and the practitioner when a common language of metaphor is found, as it not only strengthens the caring relationship, but assists in bringing the client's subjective view of their illness to the table for both to share. We both felt that the use of metaphoric language and narrative had helped us to make sense of Ann's illness and its consequences and also to integrate the experience both personally and professionally. As Richardson (1990, p. 116) puts it, 'All language has grammatical, narrative and rhetorical structures which create value, bestow meaning.'

Ann's metaphors

With my experience of cancer, I became acutely aware of the language and labels surrounding such a 'journey'. Terms such as the 'cancer journey', the 'roller coaster ride', and the 'cancer victim' were common terms within the cancer experience and circle. I felt that these terms were metaphors I would not have used to describe the reality of my experience. Frustration at not being 'heard' honestly and authentically led me to question how we as professionals within palliative and cancer care use language. My cancer experience had felt more like a 'hijacking' than a journey. I felt that I'd been kidnapped; my experience had not been planned; I did not have an itinerary nor had I bought a ticket for this experience. Nor did I have a clearly defined destination to which I was heading. The description of the 'rollercoaster ride' also felt inappropriate. Rollercoasters are something generally associated with amusement parks, but there was nothing amusing about a cancer diagnosis. I did not choose nor wish to go on this ride. There were no thrills, laughs, and exhilarated excitement. I was most certainly not going to get off the ride and think 'let's do it again'. It had felt more like a tornado, an unexpected act of nature; a fury that came in and swept up all aspects of my life and tossed them to the wind.

The experience brought lessons for us both on how important language can be in creating an authentic therapeutic relationship, and how important it is for professionals 'on this side of the fence' to listen carefully to the dialogue and description of those 'on the other side'.

Mindfulness

We had both developed an interest in mindfulness-based practice. Mindfulness is defined by the Dalai Lama as the Buddhist practice of being 'truly present' (Dalai Lama, 2001). When Ann was diagnosed with cancer, she developed a keen interest in exploring complementary therapies and practice with regard to her treatment and began to develop her own mindfulness-based practice as a form of healing. As social workers we had both had learned to be client focused and truly present with the client's experience, without judgement or labelling. It became an even greater challenge to apply this philosophy to our own situation. Turner (2009) states that traditional Buddhist mindfulness training to alleviate human suffering is compatible with social work ethics 'to enhance human wellbeing' (National Association of Social Workers, 1999, Code of Ethics).Bruce and Davies (2005) talk about the benefits of developing mindfulness practice for both the client and practitioner in working in palliative care as it fosters openness and supports 'letting go' and making space for whatever is happening in attending to living and dying. Perhaps being mindful and truly present is the way in which we cultivate true compassion in our personal and professional lives and is particularly important in palliative care, where time is so limited and precious. Papadatou (2009) describes how working in palliative care and with the bereaved helps us to experience an altered sense of time and helps us to live in the present moment with an acute awareness and aliveness. It is a place of work where 'doing becomes less important than being with' (p. 53).

Papadatou (2009) also feels that we in this work are engaged in an existential quest for meaning through suffering and its transformation. Vachon (2008) reflects on the power of the practice of mindfulness in palliative care, and feels that patients can die well only when caregivers are truly present with them. We believe that the mindfulness-based practice of being truly present provided us with a tool throughout Ann's illness and enhanced our ability to continue our work in palliative care. We also feel strongly that the greatest lesson is to listen acutely in the present moment and to listen to the unique human voice and the story to be told.

Supervision

During this time, supervision with an external supervisor, a trained and experienced social worker who had worked in palliative care and who was comfortable with high levels of emotional expression, became a 'lighthouse'. particularly for Rosemary while Ann was on extended sick leave. The 'lighthouse' metaphor conveys some of the power and empowerment that the process of supervision brought during this time.

Our supervisor had been a source of affirmation and comfort before the crisis, and monthly supervision was now greeted with even greater energy as work-related stories and reactions became so entangled. Within the domains of this private space there was the opportunity to unleash concerns in safety. Tehan (2005) outlines the importance of the need for access to professional supervision to successfully transition a workplace when an employee has a life-threatening illness, for both the colleague diagnosed and the colleagues witnessing. Kadushin (1992) identifies a model of social work supervision which has three functions: administrative, educational, and supportive. Within our organization, practitioners were offered internal supervision from their line manager as well as the option to engage an external supervisor more specific to their disciplines. The internal supervisor dealt with the administrative aspects that ensured that we were working within the organization's structures to obtain the best outcome for the client and meet the strategic goals of the agency. Internal supervision also provided for the educational function and professional development, exploring work practice and identifying gaps in our skills base and practice (Kadushin, 1992, p. 20). However, external supervision had become for both of us the 'lighthouse', as it was here that we were able to receive support and encouragement. It focused more on the emotional experience of the practitioner working in a palliative care setting and helped to improve morale and job satisfaction (Kadushin, 1992). The 'lighthouse' had provided opportunities for the sharing of the richness and depth of our storytelling over the years.

Conclusion

We believe that a narrative approach is essential in examining issues related to caregiver stress and staff support when a team member is diagnosed with a life-threatening illness. It allows for the exploration of stresses within the personal and professional realm of experience and for the discovery of what is most helpful in such circumstances. It is important to state that these are our own unique experiences and reflections based on our personal and professional histories and styles, our collegial relationship, and workplace setting. What emerged through close examination of the experiences we have described was the value we placed on the shared understanding of social work practice within palliative care, our common language, our use of professional supervision, and perhaps most importantly the compassion of our leader at the time. Above all we would like to emphasize the importance of organizational policy and practice that is committed to upholding staff well-being as well as striving to meet clients' needs: in other words, an organization committed to the cultivation of compassion for those on both side of the fence.

References

Baldwin, D.C. (1994). The role of interdisciplinary education & teamwork in primary care & health care reform. Rockville, MD: Health Resources and Services Administration, Bureau of Health Professions.

Bottomley, J. (2009). What's Love got to do with it? Grief in Australian workplaces. *Grief Matters, Australian Journal of Grief and Bereavement*, **12**(3).

Bottomley, J. and Tehan, M. (2005). 'They don't know what to say or do!': A research report on developing a best practice support model in the workplace for people with a life-threatening illness and employed carers. Palliative Care Victoria, Australia.

Bowman, T. (2009). A cruse of hope. In *Voices of Cruse: 1959–2009*. Richmond, UK: Cruse Bereavement Care.

Bruce, A. and Davies, B. (2005). Mindfulness in hospice care: Practising meditation in action. *Qualitative Health Research*, **15**(10), 1329–44.

Catkins Keidel, G. (2002). Burnout and compassion fatigue among hospice caregivers. *American Journal of Hospice and Palliative Care*, **19**(3).

Charles-Edwards, D. (2009). Empowering people at work in the face of death and bereavement. *Death Studies*, **33**(5), 420–36.

Coupland, P. and Raphael, B. (2009). Editorial: Grief matters. *Australian Journal of Grief and Bereavement*, **12**(3).

Dalai Lama, *The Art of Living*, Thorsons, Harper Collins Publishers, London, 2001.

Dickinson, E. (1959). The Selected poems of Emily Dickinson, ed. James Reeves. London: Heinemann Educational.

Doka, K. (1989). *Disenfranchized Grief: Recognizing Hidden Sorrow*. New York:Lexington Books.

Frank, A.W. (1995). *The Wounded Storyteller: Body, Illness and Ethics*. Chicago: University of Chicago Press.

Gunaratam, Y. and Oliviere, D. (eds) (2009). *Narratives and Stories in Health Care: Illness, Dying, and Bereavement*. Oxford: Oxford University Press.

Halifax, Joan (1995). *Being with Dying: Contemplative Approaches to Working with Dying People*. Project on Being With Dying (Death In America Project). Upaya, NM: Upaya Buddhist Organisation.

Halifax, Joan (2008). *Being with Dying: Cultivating Compassion and Fearlessness in the Presence of Death*. Boston: Shambala.

Kadushin, A. (1992). *Supervision in Social Work*, 3rd edn. New York: Columbia University Press.

Kauffman, S.A. (1995). *At Home in the Universe: the Search for Laws of Self-Organizaion & Complexity*, Oxford: Oxford University Press.

Ovretveit, J. (1996). Five ways to Describe a Multidisciplinary team, *Journal of Interproffessional Care* **10**(2), 162–72.

Papadatou, D. (2009). *In the Face of Death: Professionals Who Care for the Dying and the Bereaved*. New York: Springer.

Penson, Richard T., Schaperia Lydia, Daniels Kristy J., Chabner Bruce A., Lynch Jnr Thomas J. (2004), Cancer as Metaphor, *The Oncologist*. Alpha Med. Press, JCO online, **9**(6), 708–16.

Reisfield & Wilson (2004), *Journal of Clinical Oncology. Official Journal of Americal Society of Clinical Oncology*, Highwire Press, JCO Online, **22** (19), 4024–7.

Richardson, L. (1990). Narrative & Sociology, *Journal of Contemporary Ethnography*, Sage Publications Inc, **19**(1), 116–135.

Rinopache, Sogyale (ed. Gayyney P. & Harvey A.) (1992). *The Tibetan Book of Living and Dying*. Random House UK Ltd.

Saville, A. (2010). *Jumping the Fence, Illness, Crisis and Loss-Voices*, Baywoood Publishing Co. Inc., **18**(3), 269.

Tehan, M. (2005). A Literature Report on developing a Best Practice Support model for Life threatening Illness in the Workplace *Palliative Care Victoria*.

Turner, Keilty, (2009) Mindfullness-The Present Moment in Social work, *Clinical Social Work Journal*, **39**: 95–103.

Vachon, Mary, ABC Stateline SA, Radio Interview (with Ian Henschke), transcript, Australia 31/10/2008.

Wolfelt, A. (2005). Healing Grief at Work: After your Workplace is Touched by Loss, Fort Collins, CO: Companion Press.

Youngson, Robin, Dr. (2006). Hummanity and Compassion In the Practice of Medicine, Holistic Health Care perspectives, Edited by professor Marc Cohen, AIMA 2006 International Holistic Helath Conference proceedings, AIMA Inc., South Melbourne, Vic., Australia.

Chapter 7

The challenge of staff support in hospice care in Zimbabwe

Val Maasdorp

No Man is an Island

No man is an island entire of itself; every man
is a piece of the continent, a part of the main;
if a clod be washed away by the sea, Europe
is the less, as well as if a promontory were, as
well as any manner of thy friends or of thine
own were; any man's death diminishes me,
because I am involved in mankind.
And therefore never send to know for whom
the bell tolls; it tolls for thee.

(John Donne (O'Malley and Thompson, 1976))

Palliative care in Zimbabwe: how it started

In 1979 Africa's first hospice was born. Island Hospice and Bereavement Service
(Island) offered a home-based palliative and bereavement care service to what is now
known as Harare in Zimbabwe. It derived its name from the poem by John Donne.

Most of the dedicated professionals and volunteers who provide service in the arena
of palliative and bereavement care regard it as a vocation rather than a 'job', despite,
or possibly because of, the unique balance of stresses and rewards.

In line with the theme of this book, which examines 'caregiver stress and staff support in illness, dying and bereavement', this chapter explores how the staff of Island
have endured, survived, and possibly even thrived in the face of the pressures of working in this field, compounded by the additional countless country-specific challenges
encountered during the three decades that Zimbabwe and Island Hospice have been
in existence.

As the original hospice in Africa, the service faced the difficulties common to all
those ground-breaking pioneers attempting to introduce the hospice concept. Island's
medical director of almost 30 years writes that 'They met variously with gratitude, support, resistance and hostility; the early years were never easy' (Williams, 2000, p. 225).

A year after Island's establishment, the nation of Zimbabwe achieved independence.
To this day some of the bereavement referrals originate from losses suffered during
the war that preceded that milestone, and that had lasted for thirteen years.

Island began as it has continued, offering a non-fee-paying home based palliative and community bereavement care service that is secular in its provision. 'But the name, unlike so many of those in England, was deliberately without religious connotation, for ahead lay the challenge of grafting hospice principles onto a multicultural society' (Williams, 2009, p. 2).

Island Hospice today

Having started life with one nurse and one part-time social worker-cum-receptionist, just over thirty years later, Island employs two medical doctors, twelve nurses, and six social workers, and has approximately 1,000 registered patients at any time.

Island presently provides direct-service palliative and bereavement care, palliative care clinics centrally located in certain communities where difficult terrain restricts vehicular access to homes, and group work with the bereaved and HIV infected. Nationally and regionally regarded as a centre of excellence, it provides a myriad training and mentorship programmes that are facilitated by clinical staff who are therefore experience-based trainers. Training courses are tailor made for health professionals, pastors, non-governmental organizations, schools, regional government health services, etc. One of the pioneer initiatives of this past decade has been in working with those children who find themselves the primary carer of a seriously ill relative.

The impact of AIDS

Whilst initially the majority of patients were cancer sufferers, in 1987 Island's first AIDS patient was registered. The subsequent and enduring pandemic has inevitably shaped the organization in many ways. Service development was tailored to encompass the particular issues that arise from an illness that has a very complex physical and emotional impact. With AIDS there is more complex denial than in cancer, as well as stigmatization, family secrecy, counselling of family members who may themselves also be infected, multiple bereavements, despair at poor availability of antiretroviral treatment, and many more symptoms to treat. With a far less predictable 'illness trajectory' than cancer, AIDS patients might experience sudden miraculous improvements when an opportunistic infection (OI) is treated, leaving staff feeling foolish if they have been preparing a family for death.

Amongst the Island staff, as the extraordinary level of national infection rate became apparent, uncertainty and fear both in terms of clinical susceptibility and personal vulnerability required constant acknowledgement and support (Maslach, 1978, and Burger, 1988, as cited in Burger, 1995, p. 34).

Initially, therefore, as Island staff were developing their HIV/AIDS knowledge and expertise, an organizational policy set a limit on the number of AIDS patients to be registered. This became redundant over a short period of time as adequate confidence and skills were acquired, and patient referrals in fact gathered momentum more slowly than expected. In addition, Kaposi's sarcoma, an AIDS-related cancer, rapidly became the most common cancer in the country, and so the AIDS/cancer distinction became less of an issue.

Record inflation and poverty: the practicalities of survival

> By the end of the 1980s, around 10 percent of the adult population was thought to be infected with HIV. This figure rose dramatically in the first half of the 1990s, peaking at more than 36 percent between 1995 and 1997. (USAID, 2008)

Zimbabwe has held several unwanted world records. In 2006 it had the lowest life expectancy rate for females at 34 years of age; one of the worst HIV epidemics 'approximately one in five adults'(UNAIDS 2006) and the highest inflation rate in the world.

In 2007 inflation was pegged at more than 14,000 per cent, with unemployment at more than 80 per cent. The proportion of the population living below the official poverty datum line had more than doubled since 2000 to an estimated 80 per cent of the total population. Zimbabwe was suffering a severe scarcity of basic commodities, such as fuel, foodstuffs, and housing, and shortages of foreign currency. Standards of service at most hospitals and clinics were decaying, the professional 'brain drain' was increasing, and infrastructure was collapsing. With a foreign currency shortage, the government found it difficult to meet costs of maintaining roads, communications, irrigation equipment, water and sewerage systems, and traffic lights, among many others (Mass Public Opinion Institute Zimbabwe, 2008).

In June 2008 state media reported that Zimbabwe's annual inflation rate had soared to 11.2 million per cent. However, independent economist John Robertson said the actual figure could be much higher. 'The figure which has been released by the Central Statistics Office is an understatement. The actual figure could be as high as 40 million per cent in June' (ZWNEWS, June 2008).

In November 2008 the practicalities of survival had become extreme, with most families unable to access sufficient food to feed themselves. The dire shortage of food became an additional stress on the staff, as patients were in no mood for counselling when they were literally starving.

'Inflation levels in Zimbabwe are running at 13.2 billion per cent a month and could reach an all-time world record within weeks. The latest figures put the country's annual rate at 516 quintillion per cent—516 followed by 18 zeros. Zimbabwean prices are currently doubling every 1.3 days' (ZWNEWS, Nov. 2008).

The consequence of this for Zimbabweans was that they must spend all available money as soon as possible before it lost its value. Staff would spend part of each day in a bank queue to withdraw their salaries, bit by bit, as the central bank placed limits on daily account withdrawals. This paltry amount would purchase 'the equivalent of the cost of one small loaf of bread a day' (ZWNEWS, Nov. 2008).

An article in the December 2008 issue of the financial magazine *Forbes Asia* put Zimbabwe's annual inflation rate at around 6.5 quindecillion novemdecillion per cent—65 followed by 107 zeroes (IRIN, March 2008).

In the years leading up to February 2009 when Zimbabwe abandoned the Zimbabwe dollar and adopted the American dollar as its currency, the creation of new bank notes was a regular occurrence. (The highest denomination bank note was the world's first 100-trillion-dollar note, which made its appearance and held value for roughly 2 weeks in January 2009 (BBC, 2010)). In order to cope with the hyperinflation and resultant free-fall of the Zimbabwean currency into oblivion, zeroes would be dropped overnight. A total of 25 zeroes were removed between August 2006 and

February 2009 (Harvard International Review, n.d.). Salaries had for some time been part paid in fuel coupons and food which had all but disappeared from shop shelves.

Optimum effectiveness as a home care team was severely hindered during this period due to fuel shortages. With all 15 Island cars queued up optimistically at a fuel station, during the 7–8 hour wait clinical supervision and case discussions would take place. Many a staff member also had to make use of medical equipment (such as bedpans) during these fuel queues.

Political tension

Apart from the economic woes being experienced, the political environment was also tense, with four contested elections being held over a period of eight years. With political polarization apparent in every aspect of community life, staff were affected in terms of their personal lives. Also, 'no go' areas obstructed their ability to visit and care for ill patients, or provide scheduled training courses.

In addition to bereavement overload due to the many deaths, the variety of losses experienced by Zimbabweans during this period has been immense. The brain drain that has depleted Zimbabwe of a significant number of professionals has impacted not only on the delivery of healthcare but also families, the overall structure of society, and thereby the support system of staff, patients, and the bereaved. Family structures, roles, generational expectations, and dreams for the future changed. Assumptions regarding reliability, sustainability, and trust in institutions such as banks, schools, and those responsible for law and order was lost.

Island Hospice: To be or not to be resilient

The question therefore poses itself: within such a social context how does an organization support its staff to carry the burden of emotionally charged palliative care work?

Considering the immense out-of-work pressures is it still possible to 'retain our humanity and be sensitive to someone else's suffering without losing ourselves in that suffering?' (de Hennezel, 1998, p. 56).

Organizational strategy

Staff support within the organization is managed both formally and informally. When Island built its own offices in 2003, it was decided to create two communal team rooms based on area of service delivery. These were initially welcomed by the nursing staff but not by the social workers. Traditionally, Island had a separate nursing department which resided in a large team-room with the attendant impromptu case discussions, whilst the social work team had individual offices allowing privacy for counselling phone calls and sessions. It was decided to combine the departments into one Community team headed by a senior social worker, in order to further improve the collaborative patient work. (Whilst social workers traditionally take on bereavement follow-up after a patient has died, Island nurses make at least one follow-up bereavement visit to effect a sense of closure for both the family and the nurse.) Providing separate counselling rooms and combining disciplines into one room achieved improved teamwork with families, but also boosted the interdisciplinary effect of informal staff support. This supports research concluding that the 'most important source of support was informal in nature with colleagues' (White et al., 2004). Timely debriefing is extremely valuable as it cannot be assumed that staff will always be sufficiently self-aware to know when they are in trouble. 'The type, timing, and level of social support available and/or accessible to affected individuals and groups may determine outcomes' (Almedom, 2004, cited in Almedom, 2005, p. 254).

In terms of the daily management of the clinical team, two nurses and a social worker are the Community team coordinators. 'The strength of any palliative care team is dependent upon its multidisciplinary effectiveness and it is reported that the best teams are those that are led from a multidisciplinary standpoint' (Hockley, 1997, cited in Macleod and Schumacher, 1999, p. 195).

The clinical team has always had a high ratio (1:2) of social workers to nurses due to its strong belief in a truly multidisciplinary approach, and its additional community bereavement service where the deceased was not a patient within our palliative care programme. There is also good racial and gender balance.

Education, clinical supervision, and meetings are aspects of Island's formal support system. Many writers have emphasized the importance of education and training in staff support (Graham et al., 1996; Ablett and Jones, 2007). All Island staff and volunteers are required to complete the Island-customized module training in palliative and bereavement care. Table 7.1 illustrates the initial and ongoing training, and some of the

Table 7.1 Island training, supervision, and mentorship (adapted from Hunt and Maasdorp, 2011)

Module/meeting	Content	Participants
1 & 2 50 hours	All aspects of terminal illnesses, their treatment, holistic approach, counselling skills, family systems, roles of team players, working with children	Nurses, social workers, volunteers
3 25 hours	Bereavement training: grief and loss models and working approaches; different grief reactions and deaths	Nurses, social workers, volunteers
Interdisciplinary meeting: weekly	Holistic palliative care issues	Nurses and social workers
Medical meeting: weekly	New referral presentations, complex cases, death reports	Nurses and social workers; medical director leads
Clinical social workers meetings: monthly	Case presentation for discussion with enhanced learning on specific issues	Social workers and voluntary attendance by nurses
Supervision: monthly	Identified problem areas with patients and families as well as personal issues impacting work; focus is on increasing self-awareness	All clinical staff have individual time with their clinical senior
Mentorship home visits	Complex medical issues or useful learning opportunities	Medical director accompanies nurse(s)
Medical debrief of a bereavement case	Medical information explained to a bereaved client struggling with a particular aspect of the death	Medical director and social worker

regular individual and group supervision and mentorship that takes place both by senior clinicians of the same discipline, and during meetings of a multidisciplinary nature.

Multidisciplinary support groups without the presence of management have been in place for many years since Island realized that multi-status support groups were not very successful. 'The literature warns of role conflict when managers facilitate support [groups]' (McKee, 1995, pp. 203–4).

Staff loyalty

In terms of conditions of service, Island staff have traditionally received salaries that are below commercial and market rates. As a donor-funded NGO, Island runs on an extremely tight budget and it is acknowledged that the staff are poorly paid.

Contrary to what one might imagine, Island has a high level of staff retention; given the economic challenges and national migration figures (an estimated 20 per cent of the Zimbabwe population are said to have moved out of Zimbabwe to the diaspora) of the last few years this is surprising. Seven staff have been with the organization for over 15 years, having a combined palliative care experience of over 160 years, and six of these for over 20 years. (See Table 7.2.) This institutional memory has proved extremely useful during recurring periods of medication shortage and treatment unavailability. Where shortages demand both innovative ideas and a memory bank in order to 'make a plan', effective substitutes and proven alternative strategies have been reintroduced when necessary.

Island provides generous vacation conditions, both as a supplement to the low salaries, but mainly as an acknowledgement that this work is demanding, with time-off alleviating stress and promoting staff resilience and replenishment. Clinical staff members receive 36 working days vacation per annum.

As new challenges arise within the operating context of Zimbabwe, the organization attempts to be creative and sensitive to the needs of its staff. Zimbabwe is unable to provide sufficient electricity to service the nation's demand, and power shortages and load-shedding are a fact of daily life. During periods of high demand electricity to certain areas will be switched off. As the majority of staff are female and mothers, the organization work day was altered to 8.00 a.m. until 4.00 p.m., hopefully allowing those staff members to travel home and cook before the evening powercut.

Table 7.2 Years of service of 18 clinical staff

Years	Staff
>20	6
>15	1
>10	2
>5	7
>2	2

With regards to personal losses amongst staff, Island offers bereavement counselling, compassionate leave conditions, a funeral assistance policy, and light duties upon return to work. Personal losses are frequent and have a major impact, both emotionally and economically, on the lives of the staff. In Zimbabwe the extended family is both a resource and a responsibility. 'Economic constraints lead to only an ever-diminishing few bearing the burdens of the family. Hence, one will find that the "richer" family members (possibly merely those that have paid employment) are constantly called upon to contribute financially' (Maasdorp and Martin, 2004, p. 57).

In a country with an estimated HIV infection rate of around 15 per cent in 2008, many of the staff are caring for ill family members and may have taken on orphans from their deceased siblings (World Health Organization, 2008). White et al. (2004, p. 441) found that with 'events in nurses' personal lives such as a death in the family or a serious illness' nurses reported that they were less able to cope and that the 'most important source of support was informal in nature with colleagues'.

Humour as a stress reliever

Humour is a distinct and audible indicator of the ambiance in the Island offices. The ability to laugh at the latest obstacle or to bring an amusing patient incident to life in a clinical meeting is a wonderful stress-reliever. Sounds of hilarity from the team room will attract other members of staff eager to join in and receive the resilience boost on offer.

Early in Island's history, a white hospice nurse made a return visit to an elderly black man in a high density suburb, to check how he had reacted to his medications. Sadly, family and friends had gathered and she realized he had died. Keen to pay her condolences and perform the culturally-acceptable ritual, she stepped gingerly through the crowd of mourners seated on the floor and found a small table, covered in a table cloth and with flowers on it, to sit upon. After speaking to the widow, she arose to take her leave, only to discover (to her horror) that she had been sitting on the coffin. This story and the shrieking glee of the staff is the stuff that hospice humour is made of.

Island, for many years, gave the staff a small bonus in the form of peanut-butter sandwiches at morning tea time. Tea time is extremely important in a post-colonial country. Elizabeth Kubler-Ross during her visit to Island in 1994 stated 'You people are more British than the British'. However in 2008 bread disappeared from the shops and this staff treat had to be cut. The staff used both formal and informal support systems in bemoaning the loss of their cherished peanut-butter sandwiches.

Stress and resilience programme for staff

Resilience survey

As part of Island's ongoing 'Care for the Carer' programme, a short questionnaire survey was carried out in November 2009. Open questions were asked regarding what stressed, and also what nourished staff, clinically, organizationally, and at home. Each was also asked to rate their resilience on a scale of one to five, with five being the most resilient. The three highest self-ratings were from three of the longest-serving clinical staff, two nurses and one social worker, all female. White et al. (2004, p. 441)

Table 7.3 Stressors

Clinical	1. Obstacles to feeling effective, mainly in relation to larger system issues and a shortage of resources
	2. Team not working well together
Organizational	Low salary
At home	1. Lack of resources
	2. Family issues—demands of illness and death

found that one of the major factors that lessened the impact of unrelieved patient suffering on palliative care nurses was clinical experience. Due to the continuous need for creative and flexible organizational structuring and job-tasking, clinical staff rarely have five years of experience but rather five years of diverse experience. This would seem to encourage personal growth and development in terms of the resultant coping skills.

The major theme that emerged from the survey indicted that in the clinical arena stress was increased when staff encountered obstacles to feeling effective. These were mainly in relation to larger system issues outside of their control and a shortage of resources. (Palliative care medications are often in short supply.) (See Tables 7.3 and 7.4.)

In answer to the open question 'Why do you stay at Island?' the following four themes emerged with (a) and (b) being dominant.

a) Organizational values and meaningful work that make a difference to people's lives

b) Positive team dynamics and relationships with colleagues

c) Opportunity for professional development

d) Flexibility and independence in the work environment.

Nurse Faith tells the heart-warming story of her visit to a very old man with cancer of the oesophagus who was too infirm to unlock the gate for her to do her initial assessment, and collapsed just inside the gate. Her arms were too large to get through the gate to take his keys and open it from the inside. So, sitting in the dirt outside the gate, she talked him through his fears and the medication regime she passed through to him. He thanked her sincerely and pulled a piece of rope from his pocket admitting that he had been about to hang himself because of his pain and desperation.

Table 7.4 Resilience boosters

Clinical	Feeling effective in the care provided
Organizational	1. Work environment dynamics—caring, supportive colleagues and a family-like atmosphere
	2. Adequate time off
At Home	1. Good social support, family, and friends
	2. Outside activities unrelated to caring

As noted elsewhere by other authors, none of the staff indicated that the nature of the work itself was a stressor. 'Although working with cancer patients is considered stressful, palliative care staff experience similar levels of psychological distress and lower levels of burnout than staff working in other specialties' (Ablett and Jones, 2007, p. 733). 'The findings indicated that most nurses did not find their work particularly stressful, and most felt well-equipped to cope with palliative care stress' (Bruneau and Ellison, 2004, p. 296).

Collegiality at Island was seen as major source of support, contrary to another of the findings of Bruneau and Ellison (2004, p. 296). 'The principal sources of support for both groups of nurses were family and friends at home rather than colleagues at work, and most felt there was little opportunity to share experiences and feelings with their colleagues.'

In support of other authors' findings, in answer to a question about patient age groups, younger patients were indicated as predominantly the most stressful group to work with (Fisher, 1996, cited in Newton and Waters, 2001, p. 532).

Stress and resilience workshops

Following the survey, a staff stress workshop using a technique devised by Dr Sandra Bertman (1991) was held on two occasions facilitated by the author and guest lecturer Dr Carol Wogrin, Director of the National Center for Death Education, Mount Ida College, Boston. The staff were divided purely on the basis of work commitments and availability. (See Tables 7.5 and 7.6.)

Whilst arguably not at the coal face of providing palliative care, Island regards administrative staff as part of the team that is responsible for the service. In fact their views were often insightful, perceptive, and sensitive.

At each workshop, the staff were asked to draw with markers on an overhead projector transparency, a picture of their ultimate stressful day. They were also asked to describe on an attached sheet what they had drawn.

Some of the drawings were then presented to the group on an overhead projector. Group discussion about each picture was facilitated, with the anonymous artist being asked not to admit ownership until after the group discussion. Major themes

Table 7.5 Group 1

Nurses	6
Social workers	2
Admin staff	5
Doctor	1
Male	5
Female	9
TOTAL	14

(Total clinical staff = 9, plus 2 receptionists classed as admin staff)

Table 7.6 Group 2

Nurses	5
Social workers	1
Admin staff	4
Male	1
Female	9
TOTAL	10

(Total clinical staff = 6, plus 2 admin staff who are clinical volunteers)

were noted during the group contribution about what this picture evoked in each in relation to their own stresses. Thereafter most of the artists were able to speak out, own their drawings, and explain what it represented for them. At both staff stress workshops the first presented picture was not owned, later indicated as a sense of nervousness. (At the follow-up resilience workshops this was not the case, with all staff extremely eager to own and have their say about their work of art.) (See Figure 7.1.)

Artist's explanation of the picture 'I didn't give you AIDS':

'The story here depicts children who are bereaved and have been left with relatives. There are cases where you find them crying because they have been physically beaten by their guardians. For me this is the worst-case scenario. Again, we find these children

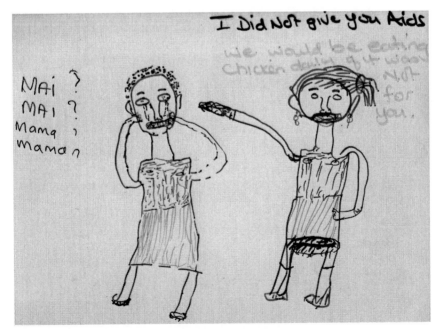

Fig. 7.1 Drawn by female Nurse (17 years with Island).
© Val Maasdorp. Reproduced with permission of the artist.

crying because a parent has died. Anything that involves children to an extent that they cry so much is too, too painful for me. Even though I know that crying is therapeutic the fact that they don't have a parent is too painful to bear. One incident was when a child was found crying at the back of the house and had told someone that: "I know that when that black car comes to take my parents they don't come back. It took my mother and she did not come back, now it is taking my father and he won't come back".

Figure 7.2, 'Nurse visits a patient who is vomiting profusely':

Initial group comments: 'many problems, vomiting, nurse leaving with a drug bag. Family feels helpless. Man with folded arms has distanced himself—not helping. Woman with arms on hips—desperate, worried. Sense of helplessness all around.'

Artist's explanation of the picture: 'Nurse visits a patient who is vomiting profusely and is in pain. Nurse has no injectable antiemetics. She asks the family to buy some while she waits. They come back with nothing because the pharmacies do not have any. The hospice nurse leaves the patient vomiting and goes back to the office to figure out what to do. She decides that she must put up a syringe driver but where to get the antiemetic. Family left helpless but said they would continue to search for the drug. Before anything works out, the patient is taken to the village to die! I as a nurse was frustrated by the fact that I could not help the patient. Patient died 2 days later having been taken to a rural area to die, but I only came to know that after 2 weeks.'

The two follow-up staff workshops focusing on resilience followed the same pattern with staff drawing what it was that gave them hope. The groups were different again based purely on availability. (See Tables 7.7 and 7.8.)

Figure 7.3, 'The support system tree':

Initial group comments: All staff observed the sun indicating that hope was shining. The tree trunk represents Island itself, and whilst different-coloured leaves and

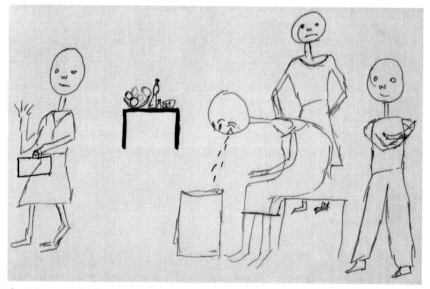

Fig. 7.2 Drawn by female Nurse (7 years with Island).
© Val Maasdorp. Reproduced with permission of the artist.

Table 7.7 Group 1

Nurses	10
Social workers	3
Admin staff	5
Doctor	1
Male	3
Female	15
TOTAL (Total clinical staff = 13, plus 3 admin staff)	18

branches indicated that at times things were tough and we might fade a little, the deep roots showed that we are anchored so we won't be uprooted. Another view was that the tree trunk represented each person with all the different challenges in life, 'some bright, some brighter'.

Artist's explanation of the picture: 'The roots of the tree show our strong support system. The black leaves on the opposite side to the sun represent life challenges, and the grey leaves in the middle are work challenges. The green represents the other side of life; the positive where the sun shines brightly. Having good roots and green leaves keeps me going strong and hopeful.'

Another drawing, made by a female nurse with seven years' experience with Island Hospice depicted a line of people. She said: 'this represents the togetherness and support I receive from the colleagues around me. We all connect in an amazing way, and the managers, those in charge, are in this with us. We are all in this together each with our different skills. There is also a power which comes from above and gives me hope.'

A 'Stress-buster' brainstorm session was later held, with staff offering ways that they themselves beat stress. There were the expected suggestions of music, dance, prayer, sharing, exercise, and the diversity of the work. The stresses of training were viewed as different to those of direct care and the job mix was regarded as playing a positive role

Table 7.8 Group 2

Nurses	1
Social workers	1
Admin staff	4
Doctor	1
Male	4
Female	3
TOTAL (Total clinical staff = 3)	7

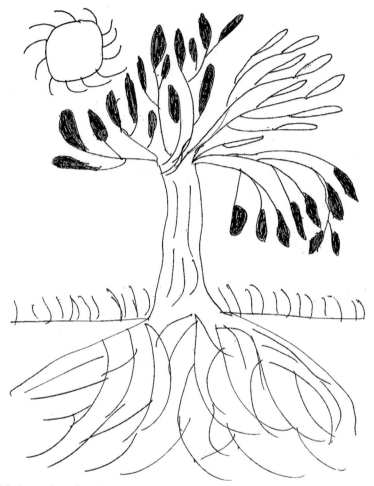

Fig. 7.3 Drawn by a female nurse (7 years with Island).
© Val Maasdorp. Reproduced with permission of the artist.

in resilience boosting. Accompanied by much humour, sex was also suggested, although one of the female nurses had earlier commented on how she was often 'too tired'. Being 'on call' at night and at weekends created definite marital strain. One nurse mentioned that her husband was always morose when she was on call for the week as it seemed that any time they decided to have sex, her on-call radio would go off.

Challenge breeds resilience

Island has a staff that appears, and furthermore perceives itself, as resilient. They have coped admirably with the ongoing daily pressures of providing palliative care in a resource-constrained environment, as well as the many years of personal challenge within the environment of Zimbabwe, a country that has faced many trials. Despite persistent years of concurrent life stressors over which one in effect can control only one's own attitude, possibly these very challenges have enhanced the quality of living.

'One turns more sharply to life with an immediacy and appreciation that would not otherwise exist' (Redfield Jamison, 1996, p. 214).

According to Rutter, 'the promotion of resilience does not lie in an avoidance of stress, but rather in encountering stress at a time and in a way that allows self-confidence and social competence to increase through mastery and appropriate responsibility' (Ablett and Jones, 2007, p. 734).

Kobasa et al. would argue that in terms of their hardiness construct, Island staff fail to have the element of control, but achieve both commitment and challenge 'akin to a zest for life that leads an individual to perceive change as an exciting opportunity for growth' (Ablett and Jones, 2007, p. 737).

Over the years this author has made observations about the characteristics of those who have thrived at Island.

- They have been well-trained and use all available opportunities to increase their clinical knowledge and 'unpick the strands of complexity in client situations' (Newton and Waters, 2001, p. 532).

- They have well-balanced personal lives and do not live solely for their work (Chochinov and Breitbart, 2000, p. 317).

- They have an ability to listen to, and withstand painful stories and not withdraw (Parkes, 2000, p. 20).

- They have respect for, and the use of, the other predominant disciplines (nursing or social work).

- They have a natural trust in and optimism about the world—despite events to the contrary (Parkes, 1986, p. 11).

Conclusion

It would appear that Island has managed to develop both organizational systems and a culture which promotes a supportive harmonious work environment, alongside the ability to use creative initiative in confronting extraordinary operational demands. Furthermore, the staff believe that through enriching the lives of others in their community their work has tremendous meaning, which compensates in some measure for the low financial remuneration.

Further research would be interesting to investigate a wider range of possible factors—including cultural and historical issues that might have helped to create the underlying sense of acceptance and fortitude. This resignation is not 'learned helplessness' (Peterson et al., 1993) but an experience based acknowledgement of forces that are beyond one's control combined with the creative energy necessary to adhere to the Zimbabwean 'mission statement' of 'Make a Plan'. Thinking out of the box? In Zimbabwe there is no box. This has resulted from a predictably unpredictable situation over the entire last three decades. Kabat-Zinn (2005, p. 248) states that 'Human beings are actually remarkably resilient to stress.' This certainly seems so in an organization of individuals in which 'No man is an island'.

I want to live
like the river flows
Carried by the surprise
of its own unfolding
    ('Fluent', by John O'Donohue (Panhala, March 2010))

References

Ablett, J.R. and Jones, R.S.P. (2007). Resilience and well-being in palliative care staff: A qualitative study of hospice nurses' experience of work. *Psycho-Oncology*, **16**, 733–40.

Almedom, A.M. (2005). Resilience, hardiness, sense of coherence and posttraumatic growth: All paths leading to 'light at the end of the tunnel'? *Journal of Loss and Trauma*, **10**, 253–65.

BBC (2010). Zimbabwe dollar sheds 12 zeros. Available at: http://news.bbc.co.uk/2/hi/africa/7865259.stm (accessed 16 March 2010).

Bertman, S. (1991). *Facing Death: Images, Insights, and Interventions*. New York: Taylor and Francis.

Bruneau, B. M.S. and Ellison, G.T.H. (2004). Palliative Care Stress in UK community hospital: Evaluation of a stress-reduction programme. *International Journal of Palliative Nursing*, **10**(6), 296–8.

Burger, A. (1995). Burnout: What is at stake? *European Journal of Palliative Care*, **2**(1), 33–5.

Chochinov, H.M. and Breitbart, W. (eds) (2000). *Handbook of Psychiatry in Palliative Medicine*, New York: Oxford University Press.

De Hennezel, M. (1998). Intimate distance. *European Journal of Palliative Care*, **5**(2), 56–9.

Graham, J., Ramirez, A.J., Cull, A., Finlay, I., Hoy, A., and Richards, M.A. (1996). Job stress and satisfaction among palliative physicians. *Palliative Medicine*, **10**, 185–94.

Harvard International Review. Zimbabwe's hyperinflation. Available at: http://hir.harvard.edu/index.php?page=article&id=1889 (accessed 16 March 2010).

Hunt, J. and Maasdorp, V. (2011). Palliative social work from an African perspective. In T. Altilio and S. Otis-Green (eds), *Textbook of Palliative Social Work*. New York: Oxford University Press.

IRIN. Zimbabwe: Inflation at 6.5 quindecillion novemdecillion percent. Available at: www.irinnews.org/Report.aspx?ReportId=82500 (accessed 16 March 2010).

Kabat-Zinn, J. (2005). *Full Catastrophe Living: Using the Wisdom of Your Body and Mind to Face Stress, Pain, and Illness*. New York: Random House.

Maasdorp, V. and Martin, R. (2004). Grief and bereavement in the developing world. In E. Burera, L. De Lima, R. Wenk, and W.Farr (eds), *Palliative Care in the developing World: Principles and Practice*. Texas: IAHPC Press, 53–66.

Macleod, R. and Schumacher, M. (1999). Hospice management—translating the vision. *European Journal of palliative Care*, **6**(6), 194–7.

Mass Public Opinion Institute Zimbabwe (2008). Desperate for change: Zimbabweans discuss the country's economic, political and social crisis, Aug.–Sept. 2007. *MPOI Report*, FGD, Aug. 2008.

McKee, E. (1995). Staff support in hospices. *International Journal of Palliative Nursing*, **1**(4), 200–5.

Newton, J. and Waters, V. (2001). Community palliative care clinical nurse specialists' descriptions of stress in their work. *International Journal of Palliative Nursing*, **7**(11), 531–40.

O'Malley, R. and Thompson, D. (eds) (1976). *John Donne: Rhyme and Reason: An Anthology*. London: Granada.

Panhala. *Fluent —John O'Donohue*. Available at: www.panhala.net/Archive/Fluent.html (accessed 25 March 2010).

Parkes, C.M. (1986). *Bereavement: Studies of Grief in Adult Life*. Harmondsworth: Penguin.

Parkes, C.M. (2000). Counselling bereaved people—help or harm? *Bereavement Care*, **19**(2), 19–21.

Peterson, C., Maier, S.F., and Seligman, M.E.P. (1993). *Learned Helplessness: A Theory for the Age of Personal Control*. New York: Oxford University Press.

Redfield Jamison, K. (1996). *An Unquiet Mind: A Memoir of Moods and Madness*. New York: First Vintage Books.

White, K., Wilkes, L., Cooper, K., and Barbato, M. (2004). The impact of unrelieved patient suffering on palliative care nurses. *International Journal of Palliative Nursing*, **10**(9), 438–44.

Williams, S.H. (2009). *The Growth of Africa's First Hospice Service: A Personal Reflection*. Dissertation, University of Cape Town.

Williams, S. (2000). Global perspective: Zimbabwe. *Palliative Medicine*, **14**, 225–6.

World Health Organization. Epidemiological Fact Sheet on HIV and AIDS. Available at http://apps.who.int/globalatlas/predefinedReports/EFS2008/full/EFS2008_ZW.pdf (accessed 28 Feb. 2010).

USAID. Zimbabwe HIV/AIDS Health Profile September 2008. Available at: www.usaid.gov/our_work/global_health/aids/Countries/africa/zimbabwe.html (accessed 28 Feb. 2010)

UNAIDS. EPI Update 2006—Sub-Saharan Africa. Available at: http://data.unaids.org/pub/EpiReport/2006/04-Sub_Saharan_Africa_2006_EpiUpdate_eng.pdf (accessed 4 June 2008).

ZWNEWS. Zimbabwe inflation rate 11.2m per cent. Available at: www.zwnews.com/issuefull.cfm?ArticleID=19362. (accessed 20 March 2010).

ZWNEWS. Zimbabwe hyperinflation will set world record within six weeks. Available at: www.zwnews.com/issuefull.cfm?ArticleID=19677 (accessed 14 Nov. 2008).

ZWNEWS. *Zimbabwe's bank queues a way of life*. Available at: www.zwnews.com/issuefull.cfm?ArticleID=19678 (accessed 14 Nov. 2008).

Chapter 8

Prevention of burnout and compassion fatigue through education and training: the project ENABLE

Amy Yin Man Chow

Background

Despite the knowledge that everyone dies, there is a general denial of death among the Chinese population in Hong Kong. As people do not talk about death, they do not prepare for it, and when they do not prepare for it, they die with unfinished business. Such denial of death may result in deep regret and severe self-blame among the bereaved loved ones. The taboo against talking about death is best illustrated by the avoidance of using the number 'four' because it rhymes with the Chinese word for death. For this reason numbers ending in four are avoided on car registration plates or in multi-storey buildings (Chow and Chan, 2006, pp. 2–3) in the belief that death may be hastened by the use of number four. Dying is also referred euphemistically as 'migrating' or 'going westward' or 'becoming a melon'. (Melon in Chinese is pronounced as 'gwa', symbolizing the sound made by the deceased at the end-of-life stage. It is a commonly used euphemism of death among Hong Kong Chinese.)

With support from the Hong Kong Jockey Club Charities Trust in 2006, the Centre on Behavioral Health (CBH) of the University of Hong Kong developed Project ENABLE (Empowerment Network for Adjustment to Bereavement and Loss in End-of-life). The project aims to educate the general public on effective death preparation and to promote enhanced adjustment to bereavement and loss.

Specifically, the Project Mission is:

a) To promote public awareness on death, dying, and bereavement.

b) Facilitate the elderly population and people with chronic and terminal illnesses, as well as their family members, in preparing for death, dying, and bereavement.

c) Develop overall competence of professionals in supporting dying patients and bereaved people.

It is the third part of the mission, the education and training of professional caregivers developed as part of Project ENABLE, that will be the main focus of this chapter. We will show that through a theoretically based and evaluated programme, training exercises that promote death awareness and reduce death anxiety can enable caregivers to work more effectively with dying and bereaved people. The name given to the training package is 'Secondary ENABLE Programme' to distinguish it from the Primary ENABLE Programme which is aimed at the general public, including both the healthy population and patients.

A dandelion is used as the symbol of the Project ENABLE. It is chosen for three reasons. Firstly, the dandelion is a plant with a wide range of uses, but is often unappreciated. Death, as the major theme of Project ENABLE, shares this similar property: an overlooked and unwelcome life event which can have lots of contributions. Secondly, the dandelion grows in different environments, including adverse ones. It has strong will power for survival. Project ENABLE hopes the participants of the project carry such characteristic after joining the programme. They are enabled and can live with strong will power. Thirdly, the dandelion has a unique way of seed dispersal. It has seed-bearing parachutes, which can be carried by wind to the ground. This symbolizes our expectation towards our secondary programme: through training the trainers, the message about life and death education can be spread to different parts of Hong Kong.

Secondary ENABLE Programme: theoretical foundation

The conceptual framework developed for the training was based on the work of several researchers and experts in the field and in particular on the understanding of stress and burnout in professional caregivers working with dying and bereaved people.

Professional caregivers are exposed to unique emotional challenges when faced with large numbers of deaths of patients and the intense grief of bereaved family members. Professionals who offer care to dying patients and bereaved families can therefore experience considerable burnout (Lyckholm, 2001; Plante and Bouchard, 1996; Swetz et al., 2009). Holland and Neimeyer (2005) named stressors such as heavy workloads, administrative procedures, and resource issues, while sources of stress that are unique in settings caring for dying patients are more often related to excessive encounters with death. Lyckholm (2001) identified various sources of stress for oncologists. These include insufficient personal or vacation time, a sense of failure, unrealistic expectations, anger, frustration, feelings of inadequacy, administrative procedures, issues of reimbursement, as well as personal grief. Katz (2006) further suggested that this stress is related to the impact of our personal selves on our professional work, described as counter-transference. Counter-transference was once considered to be an obstacle in therapy, but is now considered as a normal and inevitable reaction of the clinician, especially in intense emotional scenarios like death and dying. If carefully used, counter-transference can be a positive force in facilitating the empathetic understanding of the carers towards the patients and bereaved persons.

Emotional challenges faced by professional carers

Holland and Neimeyer (2005) proposed a list of reasons why excessive encounters with death and dying can be stressful for the professional caregiver. These include: perceived failure in treating terminal illness, confrontations with the caregiver's own mortality, death anxiety, feelings of incompetence in communicating with dying patients and bereaved families, discomfort in facing intense emotions relating to breaking of bad news, and grieving the loss of a patient. More importantly, these feelings and reactions may not be properly acknowledged and are sometimes disenfranchised because of the myth that professionals are capable of handling all these challenges.

Papadatou (2000) addressed the same issues but extended it to all healthcare professionals. She termed the phenomenon *professional grief*, which is experienced in relation to different losses in the healthcare setting. The losses include loss of a close relationship with a patient, loss of goals in the relationship when the death is impending, and losses related to professional self-image, expectations, and role. Personal grief might be related to past unresolved losses or anticipated future losses of the professional caregivers, or even the confrontation of one's own mortality. The sources of stress can therefore be experienced at both professional and personal levels. Though the former source is usually addressed by training, the latter is receiving less attention. Death anxiety, which is related to past or anticipated losses and confrontation of one's mortality, is the commonly identified stressor at a personal level.

Possible strategies in working with stressors in death and dying settings

Lyckholm (2001) suggested an array of coping strategies in facing work-related stress. Most of the strategies are related to self-care, and include frequent short breaks, extended rest time for rejuvenation, adequate sleep, physical activity, hobbies, pastimes, personal time for reflection, sharing, time management, prioritization, humour, grief work, and reading. There is also a specific suggestion about seeking a balance in personal and professional life. Self-care is also proposed by Kearney et al. (2009). Their description of Exquisite Empathy and self-awareness can be found in Chapter 4 in this book. Specifically, self-awareness is cultivated through Mindfulness Meditation practice and reflective writing. Swetz et al. (2009) have listed strategies in preventing burnout collected from an online survey with 30 physicians who care for dying patients. The list included physical well-being, professional relationships, talking with others, hobbies, clinical variety, personal relationships, personal boundaries, time away, passion for one's work, realistic expectations, humour and laughter, and remembering patients. Papadatou (2000) proposed meaning-making and loss transcendence as the two key strategies in working through professional grief.

Death anxiety as a major source of stress

In his *Death Anxiety Handbook* Neimeyer (1994) offers a systematic review of the literature on death anxiety and how it can be measured. He comments that death anxiety is an elusive term, which is sometimes used interchangeably with 'death threat', 'fear of death', and 'death concern.' In his later writing, he offers a definition of death anxiety as 'a cluster of death attitudes characterized by fear, threat, unease, discomfort, and similar negative emotional reactions, as well as anxiety in the psychodynamic sense as a kind of diffuse fear that has no clear object' (Neimeyer, Moser, and Wittkowski, 2003, p. 47).

Death anxiety, therefore, is not merely the anxiety towards death, but a mixture of feelings, attitudes, and reactions.

Tomer and Eliason (2000a, 2005) proposed and tested a comprehensive model of death anxiety. They found that three primary determinants of death anxiety are past-related regrets, future-related regrets and a sense of coherence. Past-related regret refers to the perceived unfulfilled accomplishment of life goals caused by the omission of something that should have been done, or commission of something that should have been avoided. It includes both cognitive and emotional components. The model suggests that the fewer the past and future regrets, the lower the level of death anxiety. The third determinant is the sense of coherence, which is conceptualized as the global orientation of the individual's inside world with the outside world. There are three components to coherence: comprehensibility (perception of confronted stimuli as structured, consistent, and clear), manageability (perception of adequacy of resources in meeting these stimuli), and meaningfulness (perception of these demands as making sense, and life as worthy of investment) about the self and the world (Antonovsky, 1987). Though the three components of coherence are predicted to be related to death anxiety, only meaningfulness has been found to have a significant correlation with it (Tomer and Eliason, 2000a). The perception of self as resourceful in finding meaning in life, and the sense of life as worth living are related to lower death anxiety. This model has been tested in college samples (Tomer and Eliason, 2000a, 2005) and community-based samples of older people in the United States (Tomer and Eliason, 2000b).

Death anxiety and counsellors

Novice counsellors have reported death or loss-related client problems as more uncomfortable to handle than other problems (Kirchberg and Neimeyer, 1991). Kirchberg, Neimeyer, and James (1998) further studied the relationship of novice counsellors' death anxiety and their behaviour with clients. Consistent with the first study, novice counsellors were found to have higher levels of distress in facing death-related client problems. Counsellors who perceived their personal mortality in fatalistic terms, and avoided reminders of death, had higher levels of distress when facing death-related client situations, as well as responding in non-empathic ways.

Based on this understanding of stress, death awareness and death anxiety, grief and loss issues, and coping strategies, an integrated model was developed as a basis for training and is presented in diagrammatic form in Figure 8.1.

Objectives of the Secondary ENABLE Programme

The ultimate goal of the training programme is to increase the emotional competence, as well as to reduce distress, of professionals working with individuals and families in death and dying scenarios (see Figure 8.2). Specifically, it is hoped to:

1. Decrease the death anxiety of the participants;
2. Increase the death salience of the participants;
3. Decrease the past regrets of the participants;

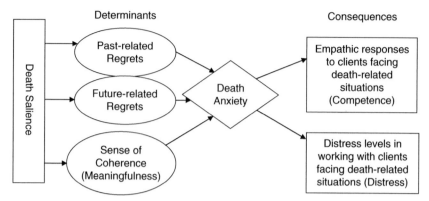

Fig. 8.1 Integrated model of death anxiety among counsellors.

4. Decrease the future regrets of the participants; and
5. Increase the sense of meaningfulness in life and work.

Components of training and camp format

The entire Secondary ENABLE Programme consisted of two components. Participants first join a three-day overnight camp. An experiential camp format was developed in the belief that working with death anxiety and regrets needs time for reflection. It was carried out in a campsite of the university, which is designated for botanical research, and was a safe place with no recreational facilities. The isolated environment provided a good space for the participants to consolidate their thinking without the distractions of their ordinary lives. The 'marathon' of three consecutive days offers an opportunity for non-interrupted in-depth reflection. Specific activities were designed to address the respective objectives. Ground rules of confidentiality and respect for individual pace of participation were agreed by all the participants. As the activities were

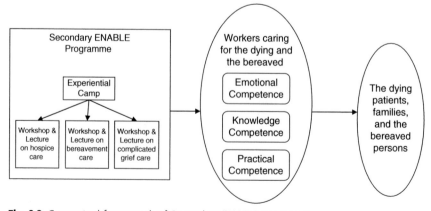

Fig. 8.2 Conceptual framework of Secondary ENABLE Programme.

emotion-provoking, debriefings were carried out after each activity in small groups. For participants who were highly moved by the events, workers were prepared to offer individual support if needed. There has been no such need so far.

Training activities

Specific training activities are designed to work on the three determinants of death anxiety as well as the salience of death stated in the integrated model shown in Figure 8.1. In addition, warm-up activities are included to open up the topic of death.

1. Visual simulation of death and ghost stories

To orientate the participants to the taboo topic of death, a slide show of different pictures and photographs related to death and loss is used as a starter. Participants are asked to view the pictures attentively and identify pictures or photographs that arouse reactions. They are asked to share pop-up thoughts, memories, and feelings in small groups. These help them to describe and explain their attitude towards death as well as their own experiences in the past. They are then asked to share about the most impressive ghost story they have ever heard. This exercise hopes to examine their death anxiety as well as their beliefs in life after death.

2. My life line

My life line is for working on past regrets. Adopting the activities of adventure-based counselling, participants are asked to walk through some obstacles wearing blindfolds. Symbolically, they are asked to review their life journey and critically examine their losses in the process of the walk. The physical obstacles in the exercise are symbols of their life obstacles, whereas the blinded situation poses a sense of uncertainty when facing loss. Debriefing is conducted to review participants' losses and their regrets in the past.

3. Anticipatory losses

The training addresses future regret through an activity on anticipatory losses. Participants are asked to prepare a list of possessions, persons, skills, and roles they treasure. Facilitators then randomly take away some of the items in the list, simulating the sudden loss of what they owned and cherished. Debriefing is offered around reactions towards these sudden losses. This pushes the participants to address the topic of future regrets.

4. Death simulation

In order to offer a greater sense of death salience, participants are asked to go through a simulation exercise of personal death. First of all, they are asked to design their tombstone, and to prepare a eulogy for themselves. A worker, playing the role of the Grim Reaper, draws from a hat the name of the participants consecutively. Once their name is called, participants are asked to go inside a big dark room, with mattresses placed in an orderly arrangement. The mattresses symbolize the burial grounds and the room a cemetery. Participants can choose to lie down on one of the mattresses, then cover their whole body with a piece of towel that they bring with them. Once they lie down, they are not allowed to move or talk, but only listen to the calling of other names, and the footsteps of others entering the room. When all the participants have entered the room, a worker leads a meditation on the dying process. The simulation ends with a ritual of rebirth and is again followed by debriefing. Their drawings of tombstones and their eulogies are put up on the wall. After the debriefing, they are asked to take a look at others' work, followed by another round of debriefing.

5. Mindfulness Meditation practice and reflective writing

Meaning-making is a process that requires reflection. Following the suggestions of Kearney at al. (2009), Mindfulness Meditation and reflective writing are used after the experiential exercises. Participants are guided to switch their attention to their body, mind, and the environment throughout the process as well as offering an opportunity for them to write down and recollect their feelings, thoughts, and physical reactions. With the written journal, participants can refer back and reflect periodically. This can prolong the effect of the exercises.

6. Lectures and skill workshops

After joining the camp, three different theory- and skill-focused workshops were offered as shown in Figure 8.2. For the workshops on hospice care, three weekly one-day workshops were offered. For the workshops on grief counselling and complicated grief counselling, five and eight weekly one-day workshops were offered respectively. The workshops included the updated research findings and theories on the topic, as well as role play on working with those who are dying and bereaved.

Preliminary evaluation

In a preliminary phase of testing and development, three points of data collection were carried out one week before the camp, immediately after the camp, and again immediately after the last workshop.

All participants in the training were invited to participate in the study. There were 7 groups, composed of 174 participants, in this phase of analysis. The number of respondents in each group ranged from 18 to 29, with a mean of 24.85. The majority of the participants in this study are females (83.9 per cent). The age range is from 21 to 68, with a mean of 37.46 and standard deviation of 9.57. Over half of the participants have no religious allegiance (55.7 per cent). For those who have a religious affiliation, Christianity was the highest percentage (19.5 per cent) of the total. Catholics contributed 16.7 per cent, and Buddhists 5.2 per cent. The length of time worked in the helping professions ranged from 0 to 40 years with a mean of 8.91 and standard deviation of 7.84.

Data was collected from self-administered questionnaires distributed by a team member who is not the trainer. Instruments used include

a. The Multidimensional Fear of Death Scale (MFODS) (Hoelter, 1979; Neimeyer and Moore, 1994): a 42-item scale that is divided into eight components. Each statement is rated on a 5-point scale with 1 = strongly agree to 5 = strongly disagree. The Cronbach alpha score is 0.75. A Chinese version has been produced and preliminarily tested. Ten items are excluded through the exploratory factor analysis. Though eight factors are still identified, the combination is slightly different from the English version.

b. The Death Attitude Profile-Revised (DAP-R) (Wong, Peker, and Gesser, 1994): a 32-item instrument to measure five types of death attitudes. It consists of a five-factor structure: 1) the Fear of Death subscale measuring negative thoughts and feelings towards death; 2) the Death Avoidance subscale measuring attempts to avoid the topic of death; 3) the Approach Acceptance subscale measuring the extent to which an individual views death as a entry point to a happy afterlife; 4) the Escape Acceptance subscale measuring the extent to which an individual views death as offering an opportunity to escape from a painful existence; and 5) the Neutral Acceptance subscale measuring the extent to which an individual accepts death as a natural reality. A Chinese version was produced and tested (Ho et al., 2009). Seven items were excluded after the exploratory factor analysis, and a similar five-factor structure identified. Since MFODS is used to measure death anxiety, the subscales of 'fear of death' and 'death avoidance' were excluded in this study. Sixteen items from the subscales and three types of death acceptance were adopted in this study.

c. The Past-regrets Questionnaire (Tomer and Eliason, 2005): which has 38 items about regrets of commission and omission. Each item is rated on a 4-point scale, from 1 = this is not at all how I feel, to 4 = this very much reflects how I feel. The items cover components of relationships, accomplishments, life experiences, personality characteristics, and life goals. The Cronbach alpha score of the questionnaire is 0.86.

d. Goal and Mode Values Inventories (Braithwaite and Law, 1985): inventories include 12 statements of life goals, which are separated into three components of cultivating relationships, pursuing spirituality, and pursuing status, respectively. They have been adopted by Tomer and Eliason (2005) as a tool for measuring future regrets. For each statement, participants are asked to rate on a 7-point scale how upset they would be if something occurred that prevented them from reaching the goal stated. The Cronbach alpha score of this inventory is 0.80.

e. The Sense of Coherence (SOC) scale (Antonovsky, 1993): a semantic differential questionnaire with 29 items (11 items on comprehensibility, 10 on manageability, and 8 on meaningfulness). Each item consists of a 7-point semantic differential scale with two anchoring phrases. The Cronbach alpha score of this scale ranged from 0.70 to 0.95.

f. Distress and competence in working with clients facing death-related situations: four items on a scale range from 0 to 10 are designed to measure the competence and distress.

Summary of findings

While unable to include a detailed summary of the findings in this chapter due to space limitations, the author would be pleased to provide further information on request via email: chowamy@hku.hk.

Significant increases in comfort and competence levels in working with both the dying and bereaved as a result of the ENABLE training programme were clearly demonstrated and are presented in the Tables 8.1 and 8.2.

The findings also indicate that the training has an effect on the death anxiety of the participants. The camp has significantly reduced the death anxiety arising from the natural fear of death as well as that related to personal and family concerns. The knowledge input of the lectures and workshops which included information about the dying process, the moment of death, and the needs of dying patients, increased participants' understanding of all of these aspects. Death anxiety related to fear of the conscious death moment, the dying process, and medical procedures was substantially reduced. However, working on unfinished business takes time, and although participants gained awareness of their unfinished business, they had to make use of the time after the camp to complete some of this work. Thus a delayed rather than an immediate effect was observed.

Tomer and Eliason's (2000a, 2000b) model suggested that death anxiety is related to life attitude, especially the dimension of meaningfulness, past-related regrets, and future-related regrets. For a better understanding of what causes the change in death anxiety, a further examination of changes in life attitudes and regrets was carried out.

Participants reported significant changes in all three dimensions of life attitudes after the workshop, but not after the camp. As change of life attitudes needs time, this result would seem to be reasonable. The participants showed better comprehension towards life, better manageability towards life, and found more meaning in their life after joining the training programme. Unlike other outcomes, there were no significant changes in the four dimensions of regrets: past-related regrets, future-related regrets (cultivating relationships), future-related regrets (pursuing knowledge), and future-related regrets (new experiences). The insignificant changes might be explained by the fact that some of the regrets cannot actually be worked through within a matter of weeks.

Table 8.1 *T*-values comparing means of comfort and competence scores over different time slots (N = 156)

	T value ($T_1 - T_2$)	*T* value ($T_2 - T_3$)	*T* value ($T_1 - T_3$)
Comfort level in working with the dying	−5.07**	−3.77**	−7.84**
Comfort level in working with bereaved persons	−4.85**	−3.34**	−7.00**
Competence level in working with the dying	−4.97**	−5.78**	−9.28**
Competence level in working with bereaved persons	−3.50**	−5.12**	−7.92**

(* $p < 0.05$,** $p < 0.01$)

Table 8.2 *d*-values comparing means of comfort and competence scores over different time slots (N = 157)

	d value (T$_1$ – T$_2$)	*d* value (T$_2$ – T$_3$)	*d* value (T$_1$ – T$_3$)
Comfort level in working with the dying	0.39	0.26	0.65
Comfort level in working with bereaved persons	0.32	0.22	0.52
Competence level in working with the dying	0.38	0.39	0.75
Competence level in working with bereaved persons	0.28	0.37	0.64

Qualitative feedback

Aside from the quantitative data collected from the questionnaires, participants were invited to share their feedback verbally in the last part of the workshop. Reported changes at personal, family, and work levels were obtained. The feedback included information about their personal, familial, and professional lives. At a personal level, participants said that they were having better emotional regulation and had more patience with others. Their stubbornness was reported to be reduced. They perceived themselves as having more energy to work after the training, though paradoxically they should have been exhausted after the camp and intensive training. Inspired by the repeated emphasis on importance of self-care, participants reported having higher self-awareness on self-care. Some participants have since turned this awareness into concrete behaviours of self-care as well. Some participants reported having some advancement in their spiritual life and felt closer to their God.

At the family level, participants reported that they treasured time with their family members more. The phrase 'I don't want to regret . . .' was mentioned frequently, though the quantitative measurements did not capture changes in these dimensions of regret. They initiated more communication with their loved ones. A few participants mentioned that they actually shared the programme and even their reflective journals and the eulogy with their loved ones. More actions to express love were carried out. Specifically, one member shared that he went to his wife's workplace immediately after the camp to pick her up. His wife was surprised and touched as the husband hadn't done this since they got married. This act reminded them of the romance they had when they were dating. Stories of facilitating reconciliation among family members were shared too. Some of them could not carry out actions because of the short duration of the training. They shared plans for family trips and family gatherings instead. All these are actually geared towards the prevention of future regrets. Participants were more comfortable with their feelings of lack of control in the counselling process, resulting in more patience and active listening towards the patients. Moreover, they reported having higher sensitivity towards the needs of their clients.

Conclusion

From both the quantitative and qualitative data, the Secondary ENABLE Programme is so far considered to be successful in meeting its objectives. The programme can help to increase the comfort and competence level of the participants in working with dying and the bereaved persons. Some dimensions of death anxiety were found to have decreased, whereas two dimensions of the death acceptance of the participants increased. Perceived meaningfulness of life has been improved at the same time. The changes in dimensions of regrets were in the direction expected, though they did not reach the statistically significant levels. Despite this non-significance in quantitative data, regrets were frequently addressed in the qualitative data. As I have already suggested, time is a crucial factor in working with regrets. Given that the length of training is relatively short, from 54 hours for the hospice care group to 94 hours for the complicated grief group in total, it is noteworthy that so many changes were reported by participants.

The evaluative study has some limitations. By adopting a multi-group pre-post test design, the examination of a lasting or delayed effect is ignored. The lack of a comparison group, or more rigorously a control group, does not allow for differentiation between the general effect of the training programme and its specific components. Sampling is another issue as the participants are all self-selected to join the programme. In order to show their gratitude to the trainer, they might report more positive changes. Efforts have been made to minimize this effect through using an independent researcher in collecting the questionnaires and explaining the importance of accuracy. Further evaluation after a 6-month interval is planned in the future.

The programme is the first of its kind in Hong Kong, developed to address the needs of Chinese professional caregivers in the field of death and dying. Its development is based on a sound theoretical foundation and has been evaluated by systematic observation. Encouragingly, it has so far been found to be effective. While addressing the professional needs of the caregivers through knowledge and skills transfer, this programme also addresses an area that has received less attention, the personal level. In view of the advancement of medical technology and an aging population, there will be more demands on professionals who care for the dying and the bereaved. It is hoped that the programme can support professional caregivers as well as being used and tested in other parts of the world with different ethnic groups.

Acknowledgements

The project described in this chapter was supported by a grant from Hong Kong Jockey Club Charitable Trust. The author would also like to express her sincere gratitude to Irene Renzenbrink for editing the chapter, Prof. Cecilia Chan, Ms Agnes Tin, Dr Grace Cheung, and Dr Wallace Chan for the partnership in developing Project ENABLE.

References

Antonovsky, A. (1987). *Unraveling the Mystery of Health*. San Francisco: Jossey-Bass.

Antonovsky, A. (1993). The structure and properties of the sense of coherence scale. *Social Science and Medicine*, **36**(6), 725–33.

Braithwaite, V.A. and Law, H.G. (1985). The structure of human values: Testing the adequacy of the Rokeach Value Survey. *Journal of Personality and Social Psychology*, 21, 203–11.

Centre on Behavioural Health, the University of Hong Kong (2010). Background of Project ENABLE. Available at www.enable.hk/enable/tch/project_enable/aboutproject/about_bg. aspx (accessed 21 May 2010).

Chow, A.Y.M. (2010). *Euphemisms of Death*. MS in preparation.

Chow, A.Y.M. and Chan, L.W.C. (2006). Introduction. In C.L.W. Chan and A.Y.M. Chow (eds), *Death, Dying and Bereavement: A Hong Kong Chinese Experience*. Hong Kong: Hong Kong University Press, 1–11.

Cohen, J. (1988). *Statistical Power for the Behavioral Sciences*, 2nd edn. Hillsdale, NJ: Erlbaum.

Ho, A.H.Y, Chan, C.L.W., Chow, A.Y.M., et al. (2009) Psychometric properties of the Chinese version of the death attitude profile-revised: DAP-R. Submitted MS.

Hoelter, J.W. (1979). Multidimensional treatment of fear of death. *Journal of Consulting and Clinical Psychology*, 47, 996–9.

Holland, J.M. and Neimeyer, R.A. (2005). Reducing the risk of burnout in end-of-life care settings: The role of daily spiritual experiences and training. *Palliative and Supportive Care*, 3, 173–81.

Huynh, T., Alderson, M., and Thompson, M. (2008). Emotional labour underlying caring: An evolutionary concept analysis. *Journal of Advanced Nursing*, 64(2), 195–208.

Katz, R.S. (2006). When our personal selves influence our professional work: An introduction to emotions and countertransference in end-of-life care. In R.S. Katz and T.A. Johnson (eds), *When Professionals Weep: Emotional and Countertransference Responses in End-of-life Care*. New York: Routledge, 3–9.

Kearney, M.K., Weininger, R.B., Vachon, M.L.S., Harrison, R.L., and Mount, B.M. (2009). Self-care of physicians caring for patients at the end of life: 'Being connected . . . A key to my survival'. *Journal of the American Medical Association*, 301(11), 1155–64.

Kirchberg, T.M. and Neimeyer, R.A. (1991). Reactions of beginning counselors to situations involving death and dying. *Death Studies*, 15, 603–10.

Kirchberg, T.M., Neimeyer, R.A., and James, R.K. (1998). Beginning counselors' death concerns and empathic responses to client situations involving death and grief. *Death Studies*, 22, 99–120.

Lyckholm, L. (2001). Dealing with stress, burnout, and grief in the practice of oncology. *Lancet Oncology*, 2, 750–5.

Neimeyer, R.A. (1994). *Death Anxiety Handbook: Research, Instrumentation, and Application*. Washington DC: Taylor & Francis.

Neimeyer, R.A. and Moore, M.K. (1994). Validity and reliability of the Multidimensional Fear of Death Scale. In R.A. Neimeyer (ed.), *Death Anxiety Handbook: Research, Instrumentation, and Application*. Washington DC: Taylor & Francis, 103–19.

Neimeyer, R.A., Moser, R.P., and Wittkowski, J. (2003). Assessing attitude towards dying and death: Psychometric considerations. *Omega Journal of Death and Dying*, 47(1), 45–76.

Papadatou, D. (2000). A proposed model of health professionals' grieving process. *Omega Journal of Death and Dying*, 41(1), 59–77.

Plante, A. and Bouchard, L. (1996). Occupational stress, burnout, and professional support in nurses working with dying patient. *Omega Journal of Death and Dying*, 32(2), 93–109.

Swetz, K.M., Harrington, S.E., Matsuyama, R. ., Shanafelt, T.D., and Lyckholm, L.J. (2009). Strategies for avoiding burnout in hospice and palliative medicine: Peer advice for physicians on achieving longevity and fulfilment. *Journal of Palliative Medicine*, **12**(9), 773–7.

Tomer, A. and Eliason, G. (2000a). Attitude about life and death: Toward a comprehensive model of death anxiety. In A. Tomer (ed.), *Death Attitudes and the Older Adult*. Philadelphia: Brunner-Routledge, 3–22.

Tomer, A. and Eliason, G. (2000b). Beliefs about self, life, and death: Testing aspects of a comprehensive model of death anxiety and death attitudes. In A. Tomer (ed.), *Death Attitudes and the Older Adult*. Philadelphia, PA: Brunner-Routledge, 137–53.

Tomer, A. and Eliason, G. (2005). Life regrets and death attitudes in college students. *Omega Journal of Death and Dying*, **51**(3), 173–95.

Wong, P.T.P., Peker, G.T., and Gesser, G. (1984). Death Attitude Profile-Revised. In R.A. Neimeyer (ed.), *Death Anxiety Handbook: Research, Instrumentation, and Application*. Washington DC: Taylor & Francis, 121–48.

Chapter 9

Staff support: a shared responsibility at Victoria Hospice Society, British Columbia, Canada

Wendy Wainwright and Susan Breiddal

Introduction

In this chapter we suggest that in order to care for patients and families in a holistic, person-centred, and grounded way, the team must have access to similar care. We further suggest that such support requires shared values, leadership, and responsibility. It is the organization's role to build policies and a sustainable infrastructure that support this care. It is the manager's role to provide leadership through human resource and clinical practices, and the employee's role to attend directly to their own needs, while at the same time being attentive to the needs of their team. Throughout we look for compassion, respect, collaboration, integrity, commitment, and excellence. We come together as equals and as human beings, focused on using our collective and individual strengths to meet and serve our patients and families at the end of life.

To this end, we offer you these three perspectives on care for the caregiver. The chapter begins with the perspective of Victoria Hospice, the organization, and how it has built a culture that values and attends to staff support. Second, we present the view of a manager who has integrated these practices in her role within her team and the organization. Finally, we present a reflection of an employee, who looks at her experiences of her work and her relationships within the organization.

> Over time, fixing and helping are draining, depleting. Over time we burn out. Service, on the other hand, is renewing. When we serve, our work itself will sustain us . . . [How do we serve?] . . . We serve with ourselves. We draw from all of our experiences. Our limitations serve, our wounds serve, even our darkness can serve. The wholeness in us serves the wholeness in others and the wholeness in life. The wholeness in you is the same as the wholeness in me. Service is relationship between equals . . . We serve life not because it is broken but because it is holy. (Remen, 1996)

So, how is it that an organization can hold and serve those who are dying and bereaved? How do we keep ourselves from taking on the tempting role of fixer or helper rather than seeing ourselves in service? We believe we do this by striving for an environment where people are seen first for their strengths and abilities, where managers work from a place of commonly held values, where leadership is shared, and where relationship and connection are key. We strive for an organization where everyone's opinion is heard and respected, where grief and sorrow are acknowledged and heard, and where differences are appreciated and celebrated. Are we there yet? Absolutely not! Do we ever stop trying to achieve this vision? Absolutely not!

Part one: the organization's perspective
History

In our community a group of people came together to care for friends and family who were dying. In 1978 they formed the Victoria Association for Care of the Dying (VACD) and were soon training volunteers to companion patients and families through illness, death, and bereavement. In 1980, when government funded a hospice project in Victoria, VACD joined this team of professionals (a social worker, physician, and nurses) to build a programme from the ground up. When permanent funding was secured in 1982, the two groups amalgamated to become the Victoria Hospice Society.

This programme has been something of an anomaly from the beginning. While it provides extensive services in the community, it also has an acute care unit housed within an existing tertiary facility. With our own board and management structure, we have sometimes struggled to find a place within our healthcare system. While maintaining our own strategic plan and policies, we have a functional partnership with our home hospital and a strong clinical partnership with community healthcare providers. At the same time, we join forces with other hospice organizations to challenge our partners and government to improve end-of-life services. Finally, and perhaps most importantly, we have the ability to fundraise and assign donations in whatever way our board and the donors designate. While approximately 50 per cent of our annual operating costs are provided and directed through our contract with the health authority, the remainder comes from our community through donations, special events, and activities. This interesting combination of support and autonomy has resulted in a scope of service and practice that goes beyond what might be expected of a relatively small organization. It has forced us to be accountable and absolutely clear about our goals and values, while it has allowed us to dedicate programme resources in a way that fulfils our mission without the usual constraints of a health bureaucracy. Staff support has been one such area.

Changes over time

Our original mission statement said that 'those providing care for the dying and bereaved have the right to receive planned emotional and spiritual support. Effective care must be co-ordinated and consistent, reflecting a common philosophy. Hospice caregivers shall have a commitment to professional and personal growth.' This speaks to the multi-faceted nature of support, acknowledging that it is the responsibility not just of the individual or of the organization but, in fact, a shared accountability between the employee, their service area, and the organization as a whole. In the beginning, as a small, 'family-type' organization, we were able to address these 'rights' in a day-to-day, personal way. Everyone attended team meetings, debriefings, and house parties, and team input on every subject was a given. We knew one another's families and many became friends. We were also part of something new and exciting; pioneers who shared a vision and a passion. As would be expected, times have changed over the last 30 years! Healthcare and hospice palliative care has changed. Resources are increasingly scarce.

Evidence is demanded as the basis of practice. The economy is uncertain. The population is aging, as is our workforce. Our programme has grown and evolved. We now have over 100 staff and 400 volunteers. Some people don't even know one another, let alone know anything about each other. Our informal attention to support was no longer serving us well. Some staff were feeling adrift from management, teams were not dealing with their issues, communication suffered, and departments and their managers came to handle support in, often, very different ways.

How we developed our support programme

Shift work, new and expanded services, and limited resources further contributed to the need to examine how we provided 'planned emotional and spiritual support'. How did we connect to one another, working within the same organization and for the same purpose? How did we keep caring for our patients and families with respect and compassion? How did we work collaboratively?

To answer these questions, we realized we had to start and end with ourselves, and in 1997 funded a project to examine staff and volunteer stress and support. It included a review of literature, a team-wide survey, interviews, and focus groups. The main recommendation of the report was the development of a formal support programme led by a support coordinator working with an interdisciplinary committee that had clear terms of reference, a work plan, and accountability to the management team (see Box 9.1).

Box 9.1 Guiding principles for developing a support programme

It is essential that staff and volunteers receive support in order to ensure the maintenance and continuing development of quality of care for dying persons and their families.

The organization's commitment to care and support for the care providers should be equivalent to care and support for patients and families.

A support programme must be:

+ formalized and structured, using planned strategies to address the needs of team members;
+ comprehensive, addressing internal and external stressors;
+ effectively managed;
+ embedded in an organizational culture that is characterized by open communication, freedom to express vulnerable feelings, and acceptance of the need to share personally stressful experiences in a supportive setting;
+ based on underlying values that serve as guideposts for the programme;
+ able to provide a continuum of strategies moving from prevention through to crisis intervention, treatment, and rehabilitation;
+ able to address the needs of the overall care provider group, yet be sufficiently diverse to meet the unique needs of individuals in the group.

(Report on Staff Support, Denis Bell, Victoria Hospice Society, 1997).

This programme was to be built on nine guiding principles identified through the literature and consultations with our team. Most importantly (see Table 9.1), it was to be a support programme that addressed the recognized internal and external stressors inherent in working in hospice palliative care (Vachon, 1995; Vachon, 1998). It required a smorgasbord approach that considered both collective and individual needs and was embedded in an organizational culture that was values-based and equivalently committed to both care providers and receivers (Riordan and Saltzer, 1992).

> *As an aside, it strikes me that a missing element in this work was the limited attention to the positive aspects of working in hospice palliative care, as reflected in the literature (Shanafelt et al., 2005) and certainly in the experience of our team. Death is expected, so not generally traumatic. People chose to do this work. Staff/patient ratios are higher than usual, teamwork is a given, and support for the care providers is part of the philosophy. Also absent from the discussion was consideration of individual and collective resiliency as an antidote to stress and burnout.*

Table 9.1 Victoria Hospice Support Committee: terms of reference

Purpose

To provide an integrated, responsive approach to support that reflects our recognition of the strengths, challenges and requirements of our staff (paid and unpaid) as they care for people who are dying and bereaved. To ensure that staff members have access to planned emotional, practical, and social support, and activities that acknowledge and address work-related needs, celebrate successes, and recognize contributions.

Assumptions

Staff support is integral to the health of any organization and requires leadership, policies, and dedicated resources to ensure its ongoing viability and success. The Support Programme does not replace the responsibility of the individual for self-care or managers for addressing needs within each department, but rather takes a broad, organizational perspective on support within the workplace. Requirements and perceptions of what is helpful will vary from one person to the next and opportunities need to be flexible and respectful of both individual and programmatic needs and resources. The activities and direction set by the Committee require regular review and evaluation.

Functions

◆ To ensure policies and procedures related to support are in place.

◆ To ensure there is a diverse programme of supportive activities available to all staff.

◆ To regularly communicate with staff regarding self-care, support activities, and staff accomplishments.

◆ To provide opportunities for networking, appreciation, and celebration.

◆ To respond to extraordinary support needs in collaboration with department manager(s).

Support Programme Components

The programme consists of the following categories of activities (each supported with a rationale and process): 1) counselling and debriefing sessions, 2) newsletter, 3) social events, 4) appreciation and recognition events, 5) retreats, and 6) educational events. The primary focus for this programme is paid staff, so our Volunteer Department has developed separate recognition activities, newsletter, and educational events. However, volunteers are included in any organization-wide social events and other activities as appropriate and as space allows.

Based on this report, the management team proposed a budget to operationalize a support programme. While the entire budget was not approved by the board, an annual amount of C$20,000 was designated for staff support. This amount allowed the creation of a formal support committee. Chaired by the Manager of Psychosocial Services, with clerical assistance, the newly formed interdisciplinary committee developed a monthly newsletter, regular recognition activities, and a calendar of events that included educational in-services, social gatherings, retreats, and support evenings. They contracted with a former Victoria Hospice counsellor to offer all employees two counselling sessions each year, at no cost. These sessions did not replace services available through our Health Authority's Employee Assistance Program, but focused on the needs and issues that can arise when working in palliative care—too many 'difficult' deaths, team conflict, enmeshment of one's own grief with that of others. While the employee's manager does not need to approve the initial two sessions, she or he is included in discussions if the counsellor and the employee agree that additional sessions would be helpful. Beyond authorizing these additional sessions, it is the manager's responsibility to ensure the employee is able to work and, if so, is supported in the workplace. Over time, the counsellor's role has expanded to include informal check-ins with the team, facilitating crisis sessions, and talking about self-care during staff and volunteer orientations.

As a committee we tried to define support for ourselves and came up with a number of views, which seem to reflect those of our broader team. Support is: 'feeling understood regarding the work you do and the context within which it is done', 'freedom to question, to be one's self, acceptance of diversity', 'mentoring and attention to supervisory needs', 'communication', 'actively promoting healing, validation of woundedness', and 'consistency between verbal and nonverbal messages regarding organizational expectations'.

Since 1997 our organization has completed several staff surveys to enquire about the impact of the support programme, work environment and job satisfaction, leadership, and a number of clinical topics. As managers, we take the results from each survey very seriously. Findings and recommendations are circulated to the team for information, discussion, and problem-solving to address any gaps or challenges identified. For example, in a recent poll the team suggested that prevention should be one of the reasons for counselling, so our counsellor now offers 'tune-ups' and self-care along with issue-specific sessions.

In our most recent survey, staff reported that their work enhances their personal life and that it is creative, provides variety, and that they have the skills needed to do their jobs. They feel their contributions are valued and that relationships within the team are good. Some concerns were also expressed. For example, a physician reported other team members aren't always willing to help them when they need it, while others wondered if policies are consistently followed across departments. In the main, people said they had sufficient autonomy, manageable workloads, and were not overwhelmed by paperwork. They want even more opportunities to process difficult deaths but find pleasure in their work and most days feel passionate about what they do.

In 2006 we wanted a way to demonstrate and remind ourselves of how we want to be with one another, our partners, our patients, and their families. Led by our Executive

Director, an interdisciplinary group worked to identify six key values (Table 9.2) and articulate what they felt to be most important about each one. The process included broad consultation and discussion until general consensus was reached. Defining our values has had enormous benefit for our team, and we are always looking for different ways to keep them visible. They appear on mugs, wall plaques, and business cards. They are a part of debriefings and difficult conversations. They prompted team training in basic Non-Violent Communication. Along with professional competencies, I use them for job descriptions, performance reviews, and reflection points within my psychosocial team.

Table 9.2 Victoria Hospice Charter of Values

Respect: We respect the intrinsic worth of each individual.

Compassion: Compassion underscores all our actions and decision-making. We demonstrate an empathic, non-judgmental manner. We believe in the power of tender acts of kindness.

Integrity: Integrity forms the basis of personal and professional practice. We take individual and collective responsibility for our actions. We are accountable and invite scrutiny. We are honest and fair in all we do within an ethical framework.

Commitment: Commitment to quality end-of-life care is fundamental to our work and our relationships. Through our dedication, we honour the people we serve, each other and ourselves.

Collaboration: Collaboration is fundamental to achieving our best work. Respectful, honest communication, with appreciation for diversity enables us to accomplish together what could not be achieved alone.

Excellence: Through the active pursuit of skills, knowledge, growth and innovation, we achieve our highest personal and professional potential in our unwavering quest for quality end-of-life care.

A final word about organizational attitudes on creating a healthy, sustainable, and respectful environment. Beyond a management commitment to communication, values-based relationships, and support, there are also other avenues or ways we encourage and promote personal and professional development within the organization. As able, we provide bursaries and funding for staff to attend educational events, conferences, and courses, as well as opportunities to provide training and resources for others. We hold team forums and updates (paid and unpaid time), and give staff opportunities to work on research projects and other activities outside the employee's usual scope of practice.

While we access the various human resource services and benefits available through the health authority, we supplement and, at times, substitute our own processes to further our commitment to being an organization that is governed by shared leadership, compassion, understanding, and consensus. The policies and procedures we most value are those addressing staff wellness and safety, support at the time of illness, death and bereavement, and patient/family care.

Part two: a manager's perspective

Strengths-based relationships

Just as stressors can arise from internal and external sources (Vachon, 2005), so too can resiliencies. Internal sources of strength may be personality factors, spiritual or religious beliefs, and learned coping strategies. External sources might include organizational structures that provide support such as supervision, opportunities for knowledge and skill development, teamwork, and job satisfaction. When I speak about organizational perspectives on support and care of the team, I speak of a shared vision that grew from our foundation, expressed in our values and implemented collaboratively. When I speak about my role as a manager of the psychosocial team, I speak with my own voice. It seems to me that we must apply the concepts we use in approaching our work with people who are dying and bereaved to our organizations, our staff, and ourselves. For me, the central concept is one of 'strengths-based' relationships. I approach people from a place that assumes they have inherent strengths and capabilities. They come into our care, our programmes, and our lives with a lifetime of experience, knowledge, and skills. We may be the experts on end-of-life care, but they are the experts on themselves. We know about diseases and medications, they know about their hopes, their families, what matters to them, and what's important.

Psychosocial care involves many pieces, but ultimately it is about helping people uncover and explore the meaning in their experience of dying. It is about making sense of their story, as they see it and they tell it. It is about holding a space so people can continue creating their story until they die; so they can die in a way that is congruent with who they are. In this, psychosocial care attends to and considers closure, grief, grief and loss, legacy, and self-reflection, all within the context of a relationship. And, all of this is defined by the person who is before us.

Leadership and management style

In doing a psychosocial assessment with patients and families I am curious about what matters to them, who they are, and how they make sense of their world, now and in the past. I want to know what they fear and what worries them, what they want from the people around them, and what needs tending to. I also want to know about their strengths and successes in life—how they got through difficult times, what strengths they draw from their relationships, their identity, or their roles. So, just as I would work with a patient or family member, so too I work with my team.

Each one of my staff brings knowledge and skills, life experiences, passion, and professionalism. They are the experts about themselves. I know they have skills and abilities, and I hold each one accountable to manage their work, their relationships, and difficult situations. If they don't have the knowledge or skills, it's not my job to rescue or fix, but rather to mentor, model, and support, in a way that reflects Remen's (1996) concept of service. Sometimes my job is easy, sometimes it's difficult. When critical feedback, 'discipline', strict instruction, or guidelines are needed, this too falls within my plan: to support each member of my team to further develop as professionals and as people.

My job is to help them discover their strengths and develop their skills, to identify and address that which gets in the way of their work, which is to help our patients and families to discover their own strengths and resiliencies. My role is to support and 'serve' them, so they can serve the people they care for. As such, we too are equals, each with our own story, our hopes, and also our woundedness (Remen, 1996; Kearney, 1997).

Staff selection

When I hire new staff, I am looking for people who have a clear sense of who they are, who have not only experienced loss and grief but who are able to reflect, with some depth, on the impact of that. Our patients and their families need people who demonstrate confidence, integrity, and openness in their relationships, people who are comfortable with the spaces between words, people who think metaphorically and can be flexible. They need to fit within our organization and department, not for homogeneity but for common values and beliefs about people and the work we do. They must be able to work independently, but also as part of a team and be able to see that the sum is greater than the parts, different and yet complementary.

I train and orient staff to learn not only about the organization and our department, but also about the theory and practice of psychosocial care, the medical aspects of our care, and the relationship between the two. Together, we identify their learning needs and their concerns. We talk about our relationship and how we'll work together, my expectations and what they might encounter during their early days in the organization and in this specialty. We talk about where they might find support, what they need to pay attention to, and then they're thrown in at the deep end and they discover they can swim!

I try to provide regular informal and formal supervision, and performance reviews that focus not only on struggles but also on successes and accomplishments. I provide a structured format for reviews but encourage individual creativity and flexibility within that. While I ask them to reflect on and demonstrate their competencies, I also ask them to comment on how I've done, how our relationship is, if they are getting the support they need, and what might be missing.

Self-care for staff

From the perspective of individual accountability, staff members are responsible for their own self-care. For me, self-care is about awareness and reflection of practice, conscious use of self, care for one's own spirit, resiliency, and coming to work well nourished emotionally, spiritually, and physically. I expect my team to come to work able and ready to be with the suffering of others, prepared to hold those difficult spaces open for what may come forth. They need to recognize that they are the most important tool they have in their work. When neglected, the result is a damaged, broken, or dull tool. When this happens people can be overwhelmed by their own suffering and sorrow, and unable to be present for others. It can take long months for someone to heal the damage in themselves in order to be able to provide care once again.

Self-care, then, requires them to work with awareness, to know their limits, to recognize their own grief and issues, and notice when they are going to be or are being triggered.

For example, knowing when your relationship with your own mother is getting in the way of how you care for someone else's mother. However, it is not enough to simply notice this; it requires people to do something with that awareness; to decide what action to take. They need strategies to deal with their issues, their grief and sorrow. Such strategies might include engaging in counselling or activities that deepen their understanding and facilitate release, finding ways to balance life and death, work and play, surrender and control, or recognizing the impact of doing such work. We can feel isolated when our own support networks, families, or friends don't see death the way we do and, often, don't even want to know about it. Our work brings the possibility of death and the reality of loss closer. We willingly engage with these aspects of life, often with a familiarity and ease that is strange or even frightening to others. Knowing this reinforces our need, not only for self-care, but also for organizational support to ensure opportunities for sharing our experiences with those who do understand.

Part three: a counsellor's perspective

Being human

This being human is a guest house,
Every morning a new arrival,
A joy, a depression, a meanness,
some momentary awareness comes
as an unexpected visitor.
Welcome and entertain them all!
Even if they're a crowd of sorrows,
who violently sweep your house
empty of its furniture,
still, treat each guest honourably.
He may be clearing you out
for some new delight.
The dark thought, the shame, the malice,
meet them at the door laughing,
and invite them in.
Be grateful for whoever comes,
because each has been sent
as a guide from beyond.

(Rumi, 1995, p. 109)

People outside the field of palliative care often ask caregivers, 'How do you do it?' 'Isn't it depressing?' These are good questions and we all have our own ways of answering them. For me, the short answer to 'How do you do it?' is that I am motivated by being in the presence of love. The longer answer is that I deal with it by recognizing and appreciating that the major requirements of my job are that I am present, that I find a place of kindness and compassion in myself, that I treat others with respect and encourage them to meet their individual and collective needs, and that I recognize the preciousness of relationships and the pain of separation. This means, however, that I am reminded every hour of every workday that I am going to die and that everyone I love is going to die. That reality is frightening and unwelcome at times, and makes me feel sad and even despairing. I have imagined myself in every configuration possible. I *am* the old woman in the bed, my grandchildren curled up beside me. I *am* the middle-aged woman watching in disbelief as her husband, who had a backache two weeks ago, takes his last breaths. It is *my* adult children weeping at his bedside. My ability to imagine my last moments, in all their sensual detail, is unending. I am sick, in pain, and afraid. It is me who will never feel the pull of the current at Stamp River, will never feel the weight of my body pulling on two fingers as I hang above a crevice, will never smell the smoky fire in my daughter's damp hair, or be alone in a meadow, or feel the cool water on my sun-warmed flesh. It is me who will never feel the waves at my feet or smell the sun on pine needles, or eat another piece of pork tenderloin, or hear the words 'Merry Christmas.' On and on it goes.

Then, out of nowhere, I am acutely aware that I am alive. I am not dying right now. I can hardly believe the joy of *knowing* that I am *here*! The people whom I love are living and breathing right *now*. I rejoice in my minor physical discomforts being just that, minor physical discomforts. I hike up the mountain and I feel the power in my legs and my heart beating strongly. I stand in the forest and I can smell the earth. I tell my husband that I love him and I mean it. I am no longer waiting for some future time when things will be different. I am not waiting for anything. When my grown children gather together for dinner, I notice. I am aware that we are *together*. I take comfort in knowing that no matter what happens from here, *no one* can take away the pure delight that I have, just . . . being . . . with . . . my . . . family.

How could I not love a job that requires me to be awake? I travel, I teach, I go to school, I take chances, I speak my mind because I *can*. I have come home. It's a good way to live life. This has been a process, and it hasn't been easy. It's still not easy. It's confusing, 'this being human is a guest house, every morning a new arrival . . . ' It has been, and continues to be, difficult to meet 'the dark thought, the shame, the malice.' Luckily, I have gradually begun to understand the workings of my inner world and to see how disconnected I can get. I see the change in small ways. I am seated in a client's home. She leans on a cane as she hobbles to the living room. I have read her chart, and I know that she is my age. I too have a limp, a side-effect of knee surgery, and I have been hoping that the limp will go away. I see her and I see myself all at the same time. Her limp is not going to go away. She is dying. I, however, have had the chance to do physiotherapy but I haven't taken it seriously. My plan to walk across Canada 'some day' just might not happen, and, in fact, the way that I am going, it will most certainly *not* happen. It is so evident that I have taken my health for granted. *Hoping* for it to get better is not enough.

> I was passionate
> Filled with longing,
> I searched
> Far and wide.
> But the day
> That the truthful one
> Found me
> I was at home.

(Halpern, 1994, p. 139)

It is clear that I have *not* been at home. In conversation with a woman on the hospice unit who is perhaps three, maybe four years older than I, the woman says, 'You know what it's like at *our* age. We don't get out very much.' What? Her words horrify me. This is not me. This is not what I want. No! I refuse!

Jon Kabat-Zinn tells us that 'our beliefs about ourselves and about our own capabilities, as well as how we see the world and the forces at play in it all, affect what we . . . find possible' (Kabat-Zinn, 1990, p. 11). I can see that what I am telling myself is what I am becoming. By ignoring the signs that my body is giving me, by not having the courage to follow my dreams, I have limited what I have found 'possible.' I have fallen asleep.

I am addicted to sugar, I overeat, and I don't get enough exercise. I watch mindless television. But I can change. I re-enter therapy; I pray; I meditate; I go to church; I read; I ask my husband to just hold me; I talk to my friends, my sisters, my children. I take up rock climbing, I run, I swim, I bike. I lose 50 pounds. I even admit to my boss that I *must* take an afternoon nap. I change all my shifts to afternoons. I make a commitment to myself that I will do *nothing* unless I want to. I stop cooking. I stop my meagre attempts to clean the house. I take those trips that were going to happen . . . when I have the money. I spit in the face of 'not getting out much anymore,' of what is 'possible.' I *feel* my strength. I *feel* my health. I have seen what it is like not to have choices, not to be able to respond to opportunity and I know that I *can* make a choice.

As I begin to reconnect to myself, I find that there is more, so much more. I am not dealing effectively with conflict. I feel irritated with my colleagues, frustrated with the organization for which I work. I get bored, then I take on too much, and I become almost paralysed with fear. My anxiety is chronic and out of control. I begin to notice my thoughts. When I am irritated or silent or start to crave chocolate I ask myself 'why?' I note the story that I am telling myself: there is blame, criticism. When I take away what everyone else is doing and focus only on my thoughts, feelings, and sensations, I am left with a stark image. I can see myself *in situ*. My behaviour has its own impact and influences my actions. It is affecting the people with whom I interact and, therefore, the interaction. My thoughts are creating my reality.

A plethora of literature talks about burnout, caregiver distress, and compassion fatigue, or uses terms such as 'death saturation,' 'chronic grief in caregivers,' or 'death-denying culture' (Jones, 2005, p. 125; Kearney, 2009, p. 1156; Papadatou, 2009, p. 122; Renzenbrink, 2004). Disenfranchised workers complain of 'toxic' work environments. These terms place responsibility or blame on vague outside sources such as 'colleagues' or 'the organization,' making it difficult to address the problem. The 'work environment' or 'the system' or 'management' doesn't exist. There is no 'system,' there are only people who work in the system. It doesn't help me, right now, to wait for someone else to change or for the 'system' to be improved. In my work in the developing world, 'systems' and 'resources,' as we understand them, barely exist. Patients are 'stacked' foot to head, two to a bed and one underneath. Palliative care sometimes means a clean glass of water, a boiled egg for dinner, or holding hands. This doesn't mean, however, that improvements aren't necessary or that services should not be evaluated in the light of how well needs are being met.

The palliative care setting is a stage for everyday drama and the palliative caregiver is automatically a principal player in the drama. The literature, however, reveals a disturbing interpretation of the play. For example, I am concerned that the literature expresses an assumption that 'dealing with death' is in itself stressful (DiTullio, 1999; Renzenbrink, 2004). 'Dealing with death' isn't necessarily stressful or unpleasant. Avoiding feelings about it, however, may be uncomfortable. By definition, palliative caregivers will continue to work with dying people and focusing on or framing our experience as being 'constantly exposed to experiences of loss' (Keidel, 2002, p. 201) places responsibility or blame on the losses rather than our response to the losses. However true it might be that caregivers experience stress, helplessly trying to fend off an army of losses marching towards them places them in a victim position. If instead I create a frame that allows me to think of my work as an opportunity to practise, over and over again, the art of being present, I will not just cope, I will thrive—as a caregiver and as a human being.

Perhaps it is time to let go of the idea that hospice care is primarily focused on death, and that our work as palliative caregivers is necessarily patient or family centred. Papadatou says that holistic care must include the experience of the caregiver, and advocates for a relation-centred approach, because of the reciprocal nature of the interactions (2009). 'If we perceive our relationships with dying and bereaved people as being solely submerged in suffering, then we neglect the immense potential for self-actualization and growth' (DiTullio, and Macdonald, 1999, p. 120). For that reason, I choose *not* to think that the purpose of my job is to relieve suffering (see www.who.int/cancer/palliative/definition/en/), because in that 'story' success depends on patients and families performing in a particular way to be relieved of their suffering. If they don't feel relief, then I haven't met my goal. How can I possibly be successful if I frame my role this way? From this perspective can I really expect to thrive? Isn't it more helpful to attempt to 'meet' whatever is there? 'The dark sobs, the shame, the malice, meet them at the door laughing and invite them in.' Wouldn't it be better to be 'grateful for whoever comes'? I think that I *can* 'meet them at the door laughing' and my health is directly related to day-to-day, moment-by-moment choices, cultivated through practice and the consistent **intention to connect**.

Jon Kabat-Zinn (1990) challenges us to 'live life as if each moment was important, as if each moment counted and could be worked with, even if it was a moment of pain, sadness, despair, or fear. This "work" involves above all the regular, disciplined practice of moment-to-moment awareness or *mindfulness*, the complete "owning" of each moment of . . . experience, good, bad or ugly' (Kabat-Zinn, 1990, p. 11). It is not that I will ever be completely successful in trying to meet my goal of being present, anymore than the person who wants to end suffering, but the difference is that in *my* story, success depends on my actions: my willingness to meet my own disconnection by thinking about why I am in conflict with a co-worker, why I don't want to visit a particular patient, or why I feel irritated with my boss. I *will* be stressed if I resist moving towards my own wholeness. When I choose to run away or avoid something difficult, I become fractured.

To live out my story I decide to *come home*, to arrive in my own experience, and to notice and accept what is happening. I must be open to sensations, thoughts, and feelings. I am willing to sit for awhile. To think, 'What do I need right now?' Then to look around me and see what is happening with others. In my story, there is a *requirement* to place value on my own way of being. There is a *requirement* to take my own experience seriously, to attend. Yes! Attend to what is happening. When I embrace both my unwillingness to face what scares me or is uncomfortable *and* my desire to be present and reconnect the disparate pieces of myself, then I practise self-care and palliative care at the *same time*. I move from trying to cope in a hostile, difficult, intense environment to beginning to thrive from the inside out.

My goal, then, is not to relieve suffering for my patients, but to show up. It's the goal, the challenge, and the reward, and I believe that it benefits the client as much as it does me, because when I stay connected to myself I am available to and present for clients. It also benefits my colleagues and, most importantly, benefits our relationships. It's the most difficult part of the job but it offers the most rewards.

Self-care in palliative care practice is the cultivation of wholeness that mirrors the holistic care that we provide for patients and families. If 'the ability to be present with respectful attention is a top priority for care providers in palliative care' and 'it is generally accepted that caring or making contact is the essential element of the . . . [caregiver/patient] relationship and that this contact makes a significant difference to the patient's sense of emotional well-being' (Benner and Wrubel, 1989; Gould, 1990; Reynolds and Scott, 2000; in de Vries, 2001, p. 507), then the principles of palliative care have been reflected in my relationships. Ideally, this is embedded in a greater system that includes the multi-disciplinary team, the department, the managers, and the administration, and all of these people who make up 'the system'. Presence and connection require people to reflect upon their experience and their own needs and to respond to the needs of the individuals, in an ever-moving reflexive loop. In this way, then there is no real separation between the concepts of palliative care and the people who deliver it. The opportunity to be present for this connection offers satisfaction to both the caregiver and the patient. 'Care-seeking and care-giving behaviours are interrelated and complementary. One of their functions is to ensure a sense of belonging to a key relationship that is significant both to the helper and to the person being helped' (Papadatou, 2009, p. 36).

This interrelationship ideally is mirrored by the supervisor/employee/colleague relationship. Ditullio and MacDonald (1999) say that in their study on coping and stress in the palliative care setting, 'support, as a hospice construct, appears to be a major reward of hospice work, and as a major stressor when perceived to be absent or insufficient' (p. 653). The organization for which I work nurtures and supports my quest to understand my own emotions, feelings, thoughts, behaviours, and ways of making meaning. For instance, in my first year of working at the hospice, I noticed that I was very squeamish about physical care and I wondered how I would deal with the sights and smells. Colleagues reached out to support me and, although I was ashamed to admit my feelings, I talked about my struggles. At counselling meetings I quickly came to realize that my feelings would be accepted, understood, and validated. I found no need to hide my frustrations, my anger, my pettiness, or my grief.

I have access to a manager, and I understand that beyond our clearly defined roles, we come together first as human beings, which mirrors my work with patients and families, where my first priority is to meet as a fellow human being and then as a counsellor meeting a patient. We are so much more than our roles as defined on paper.

And yet, I depend on my manager. There have been many times over the years that I have spent a two-hour block of time with her, simply by knocking at her door and asking to talk or by making a phone call after hours. I am reassured that it isn't a bother, and that there is time to connect. There have also been long periods of time when I felt no need check in and that has been fine too.

Having a supervisor who has been completely truthful with me has helped me to appreciate the value and wisdom of speaking clearly and directly to the person with whom I am unhappy. I am validated in my belief that 'process' is everything. For instance, if I complain about a co-worker, there is an expectation that I will resolve the issue without intervention; the supervisor is simply bearing witness to my struggle. There is room to take action or to come to an understanding and take no action. I am supported in both choices. Any attempt to try to 'fix' staff relations might solve the immediate problem, but might also damage the relationship. Process is everything.

Another example of process is that there are no secrets. If someone has reported my 'bad' behaviour I have been told clearly who reported it and what was said. Then there has been silence, or maybe, 'So what happened?' No judgement, no accusation, just, 'This is what I heard.' There is room to react, to rant, to be defensive, and then I think. I sit, I consider, I reflect. I come back to my supervisor and we decide together what happens next. There is no reproach, no punishment. It is more like a kindly desire to see me grow.

Has it been a perfect relationship? Is there such a thing? If perfect means without difficulty or conflict, then no, it hasn't been perfect. This relationship has been a shared experience with real struggles, involving my distress, not only with patients, with colleagues, or with the organization, but also with concepts of care. There have been times when I refused to show up or speak to my supervisor, times of weeping and consoling as I poured out my hurt, my shame, my anger, and other times of sharing ideas, arguing, brainstorming, and feeling joy when I came up with creative solutions. However, work is not the whole picture, because at the same time as my career has unfolded, my life has been full: my mother's dementia and death, my health crisis, the well-being of my children, my marriage, my athletic accomplishments, all the things that make me a whole person. I am not separate from my work. My relationships with my patients, my colleagues, my friends, and my family are not separate because *I* am the constant. Who I am is inseparable from my relationship with my supervisor and my colleagues and the people with whom I work.

My relationship with my manager, although satisfying, is more complex than it looks. It allows for two fully human people who can be headstrong, bitchy, stubborn, inattentive, impulsive, and reactive; two people who are sure that they are *right*; two people who laugh out loud and hug each other when it's all over. It is an opportunity to be receptive, to act on the desire to understand, to connect. It is a validation that the relationship is not just about being *only* kind, compassionate people. This relationship allows for the possibility of being *everything* we are. We just can't help being who we are! But I know that I wouldn't want it to be any other way. It has allowed us to grow as people, as we witness our own and each other's 'unexpected visitor(s)' . . . We have welcomed, or perhaps only *entertained*, them all, but together, we have 'honoured each guest' and 'invite(d) them in,' appreciating that 'each has been sent as a guide' (Rumi, 1995, p. 109). Ah yes, being human.

References

de Vries, K. (2001). Enhancing creativity to improve palliative care: The role of an experiential self-care workshop. *International Journal of Palliative Nursing*, 7(10), 505–11.

DiTullio, M. and MacDonald, D. (1999). The struggle for the soul of hospice: Stress, coping, and change among hospice workers. *American Journal of Hospice & Palliative Care*, 16(5), 641–55.

Halpern, D. (1994). *Lalla. Holy Fire: Nine Visionary Poets and the Quest for Enlightenment*, trans. J. Hirshfield. New York: Harper Perennial.

Jones, S.H. (2005). A self-care plan for hospice workers. *American Journal of Hospice and Palliative Care*, 22(2), 125–8.

Kabat-Zinn, J. (1990). *Full Catastrophe Living: Using the Wisdom of Your Body and Mind to Face Stress, Pain and Illness*. New York: Dell.

Kearney, M. (1997). *Mortally Wounded: Stories of Soul Pain, Death, and Healing*. New York: Scribners.

Kearney, M., Weiniger, R., Vachon, M., Harrison, R., and Mount, B. (2009). Self-care of physicians caring for patients at the end of life: 'Being connected . . . a key to my survival'. *Journal of the American Medical Assocation*, 301(11), 1155–64.

Keidel, G. (2002). Burnout and compassion fatigue among hospice caregivers. *American Journal of Hospice & Palliative Care*, 19(3), 200–5.

Papadatou, D. (2009). *In the Face of Death: Professionals Who Care For the Dying and the Bereaved*. New York: Springer Publishing Company.

Remen, R. (1996). In the service of life. *Noetic Sciences Review*, Spring.

Renzenbrink, I. (2004). Relentless self care. In P. Silverman and J. Berzoff, *Living with Dying: A Handbook for End of Life Care Practitioners* New York: Columbia University Press.

Riordan, R. and Saltzer, S. (1992). Burnout prevention among health care providers working with the terminally ill: A literature review. *OMEGA*, 25(1), 17–24.

Rumi (1995). The guesthouse. *The Essential Rumi*, trans. C. Barcs with J. Moyne. San Francisco: Harper.

Shanafelt, T., Novotny, P., Johnson, M.E., et al. (2005). The wellbeing and personal wellness promotion strategies of medical oncologists in the North Central Cancer Treatment Group. *Oncology*, **68**, 23–32.

Vachon, M. (1995). Staff stress in hospice/palliative care: A review. *Palliative Medicine*, **9**, 91–122.

Vachon, M. (1998). The stress of professional caregivers. In D. Doyle, G. Hanks, and N. Macdonald (eds), *The Oxford Textbook of Palliative Medicine*. Oxford: Oxford University Press, 919–39.

Vachon, M.L.S. (2005). Emotional issues in palliative medicine. In D. Doyle, G. Hanks, N.I. Cherny, and K. Calman (eds), *Oxford Textbook of Palliative Medicine*, 3rd edn. Oxford: Oxford University Press, 961–85.

Chapter 10

Leadership and staff care, self-care and self-awareness: reflections from St Christopher's Hospice, London

Andrea Dechamps

This chapter will explore issues of leadership and management practices in relation to caregiver stress and support. It will be argued that if those engaged in caring for those with life-limiting illnesses are to practise 'relentless self-care', as postulated by Renzenbrink (2004), then this also needs to be about rigorous self-awareness and a commitment to reflection and dialogue, both for leaders and their teams. This takes discipline and maturity. How as leaders in palliative care do we foster a culture open to self-care as well as self-awareness? In today's ever more complex healthcare context how do we balance performance expectations and the need to deliver against targets with care for our staff and also acknowledge the emotional impact of their work?

In writing about these questions I will draw from personal as well as professional experience, and in particular the framework for support at St Christopher's Hospice in London, UK. The term 'leader' in this context will refer to managers at all levels.

The context for staff and self-care in palliative care

Any such exploration needs to be set in context. Think of a stranger asking, '. . . and what do *you* do for a living?' For those of us working in palliative care there will be some fairly typical reactions to our reply. On occasion there will be that momentary silence; then there will be those who launch into the story of a recent family death. Many will respond with awe, maybe some discomfort. There is the implication that our work is somehow out of the ordinary, exceptionally challenging, and perhaps also uniquely rewarding. How we position ourselves in relation to this perception is an interesting question.

There is no doubt that working with patients with life-limiting illnesses and their families requires considerable personal resources. Dealing with families around the time of death can be emotionally exhausting for clinicians. Most days I hear stories from my team regarding desperately complex family situations. The direct impact on team members, whether spoken or not, is evident.

And yet, working in end-of life care is *not* intrinsically more challenging and staff stress in this context *not* more prevalent in comparison to other areas within health and social care, such as for example oncology or mental health (Sherman et al., 2006). It is crucial to contextualize work in palliative care. In Monroe's words (Monroe, 2004, p. 450), 'palliative care is not a uniquely stressful profession.'

Perhaps surprisingly, research shows stress in palliative care to be related not necessarily to direct patient work but to conflict within the work environment. Vachon (1995) reports 48 per cent of hospice/palliative care staff quoting stress from organizational issues. Barnes' literature review of stress in children's hospices (2001) highlights the main sources of stress as conflict amongst staff groups, communication issues, and role conflict. Vachon (1995) also points to the impact of broader societal issues such as the position of palliative care in the current healthcare environment.

So here we have a discourse describing work with the dying and bereaved as exceptional, extraordinary and with the implication of heroic effort on the part of the multi-disciplinary team. The public's beliefs and partly unconscious assumptions about the work of palliative care practitioners put them on a pedestal. However, as we move from the pioneering days of the hospice movement into the present there is an increasing call for an altogether more dispassionate look at these issues. Payne puts it clearly: 'Concerns about negative aspects of stress in palliative care need to be proportionate to the evidence of difficulties' (Payne, 2008, p. 248). He advocates a look at what works (rather than what does not) and argues for research, management, and professional work to focus on successful self-management and self-care rather than lingering over the negative consequences of stress. Similarly Monroe (2004) points to the successful implementation of various personal and organizational strategies as one explanation for the comparatively low stress levels in palliative care. Vachon calls these the 'buffering mechanisms' (Vachon, 1995, p. 109) for mitigating stress. Alongside clinical supervision, staff support programmes, education, and team development, self-care is crucial here.

Relentless self-care and rigorous self-awareness

So what is self-care all about? Renzenbrink (2004) explores this in some detail and adds an intriguing twist to the concept when she calls for *relentless* self-care. She herself describes the term as possibly rather dramatic. The word certainly is evocative. Relentless implies persistent effort, never slackening, continuing always at an intense level. Relentless self-care is not a soft option. It goes beyond doughnuts at team meetings, the odd swim or glass of wine after a long day. Relentless, interestingly, also carries connotations of unyielding, even grim, determination. Or, in somewhat more positive terms, of commitment and discipline.

Self-care is partly about being gentle with ourselves, taking for ourselves when much of this work is about giving. However, it is also about the responsibility to keep ourselves in the best possible shape, physically, mentally, emotionally, and spiritually.

Relentless self-care includes and needs to be matched by rigorous self-awareness. Renzenbrink refers to this when she invites readers to consider therapy and to discover their values. Self-awareness and ongoing reflection (whether through therapy or indeed a multitude of other ways) are crucial for those working in palliative care, for their own and the patients' sake. For the purpose of this chapter I will touch on two particular aspects, the confrontation with our mortality and the connection with ordinariness.

Awareness of our own mortality

Inevitably, palliative care confronts us with our own mortality. Some will actively seek this confrontation, in an attempt to make sense and find meaning and maybe also to achieve some mastery regarding their fear of death. Some may strive for the particular intensity of that confrontation as it heightens their sense of being alive, or of immunity, as a polarity develops between us the clinicians and those others who embody illness and death. Should death unexpectedly affect one of us personally (it may be a friend or a relative dying), it can catch us unaware and pierce the safe order of things we have constructed for ourselves. Of course, intellectually we know otherwise, and yet we may return repeatedly to a degree of denial as we look for certainty in an ultimately unsafe world. Yalom (2008) likens facing one's mortality to staring at the sun. We can only do so much of it, brief moments, no more.

There is indeed a fine line between a healthy denial which allows us to focus on the job to be done, a denial which is recognized as such and can be suspended, and on the other hand a denial pulled ever more tightly around a fragile and maybe terrified self. As palliative care workers we need the willingness to stand in the heat of that sun, perhaps just for short moments, but again and again.

We have a poignant reminder to remain connected with the inevitable degeneration of our own body, mind, and ultimate death in the ancient Greek myth of Chiron, the centaur who taught healing yet himself had incurable wounds. Chiron is the archetypal wounded healer who from the place of his own woundedness and suffering reaches out to others (Kearney, 1996, pp. 42–56).

Someone who teaches death confrontation (Papadatou, 2009) in an extraordinary way is Scott Eberle, medical director of the Hospice of Petaluma, California, and wilderness guide. He brings together his experience as a hospice physician with ancient Mayan rites-of-passage teaching in a programme called 'the practice of living and dying' (www.schooloflostborders.org). These are workshops that invite participants to move through four symbolic stages in conscious preparation for death. From the first stage of Decision Road (recognizing the approaching death) participants will move through the Death Lodge (the place of relationships and saying goodbye), then the Purpose Circle (the place of life review, remembering with honesty), to the final stage of the Great Ball Court (the place of transition). For those physically dying this last stage is about physical death; for those symbolically dying (the workshop participants) there is the chance for re-integration into life. Eberle's ultimate message is simple. There are lessons in the 'final crossing' (Eberle, 2006), lessons which can be learnt now. This is indeed about *learning to die in order to live*.

Whether through attendance at a programme such as the above, through reflections in personal therapy, supervision, or quite simply the daily routine of working in palliative care, death confrontation, in Papadatou's words, 'opens up possibilities and offers new choices and an incredible freedom to live differently' (Papadatou, 2009, p. 186). This is where self-awareness links closely with self-care. And not only that, such self-awareness is also an essential prerequisite for delivering good patient care. 'The lessons learned when we address our existential concerns . . . can help us assist dying and bereaved people to address their own concerns, value life, and love themselves and others with greater depth and clarity' (Papadatou, 2009, p. 186).

Connection with ordinariness

The other strand to consider in terms of self-awareness linked with self-care is the need to seek clarity with regards to *why* we do this work. These are questions about motivation and purpose. Working with the dying can be seductive, feeding stories of ourselves as somehow being very special. Those are dangerous dreams, for patients and practitioners.

As part of our growing up we all have to negotiate our development through pride and shame, between delusions of omnipotence at one end of the spectrum to worthlessness at the other, towards a secure and healthy sense of self. The challenge of staying rooted firmly in the middle ground remains a lifelong task. How do we tell the story of what has brought us to this work? Do we see ourselves as saviours, or at least rescuers? On the flip side, do we have fears of uselessness or maybe a conviction that success is undeserved? To be fair, much can be achieved from that heroic stance, but much energy will also be spent defending that persona. Being simply 'good enough' and 'ordinary' on the other hand is about healthy pride in our achievements as well as the ability to accept shortcomings and what we yet have to learn.

Translating 'connection with ordinariness' into practice, this may mean monitoring my patterns of making superhuman efforts or noticing whether I can respond appropriately to criticism. With colleagues it may mean pointing out gently when they come across as overly self-critical. Or in the team, when despite all efforts we are unable to achieve for patients what we have set our hearts on, it may mean taking time to acknowledge that none of us are invincible or indeed infallible (and staying with the potential discomfort this evokes).

Johnson, in his exploration of the narcissistic personality style, puts it extremely well: 'Once his ordinariness is realized, he can express his gift as just that—a gift. His gift is not who he is; his humanness is who he is' (Johnson, 1994, p. 165). It is from this place of human ordinariness, where real connection with others becomes possible, that those working in palliative care will be able to deliver best patient care. Also, it is from this place of human ordinariness, having let go of the ultimately impossible demands of the heroic journey, that a more gentle approach to self-care becomes feasible.

A personal story

My father was an extraordinary man. He fought in the German army during the Second World War, and despite misgivings about the regime was a committed leader of his men. He became involved at the fringes of the resistance movement; he then spent eleven years in a Siberian labour camp as a prisoner of war. He returned home in 1956 with the last men who ever came back from Russian captivity.

He was also a man who had witnessed death many times, at close quarters, who again and again had sat with those dying, who had made the care of the dead part of his purpose, and, never thinking he would make it back from Siberia, at that time had made peace with his own death.

And you still wonder how I ended up working in palliative care? I grew up with (in my eyes) a hero and an immense legacy. Shortly before my father died, almost twenty years ago, I was able to tell him that I had just landed a job in an AIDS project. His delight was palpable, his faith in me huge.

My own journey in relation to this intergenerational legacy has been an interesting one. For some years I embraced and carried my father's purpose, continuing on his heroic journey. In fact it served me well during those years. Much got done, much was achieved. Of course, living his legacy also helped in my grief for him as it allowed me to stay closely connected. Yet, it felt heavy, at times a huge responsibility. It took some time for me to recognize his legacy, bring it into consciousness as such. With time I found myself more able to distinguish between what was my father's and what was mine, what man I had made him out to be and what man he really was, how I could take inspiration from his life and yet live my own. With that, and it felt like another step into adulthood, came the gradual ability to let go of the need to be heroic.

Finding my ordinariness—what difference has it made? I know that others find me less intense these days. I experience easier and perhaps more real connection with others. I still continue to work in end-of-life care and crucially it has become survivable. Continuing on the heroic path may have ultimately led to a dead end. I walk with a lighter step. And, I find myself better able to take care of myself.

Reflections on leadership

For leaders in end-of-life care the twin responsibilities of their own individual self-care and self-awareness are closely linked with the responsibility for staff care whilst ensuring delivery of patient care. For a moment let us consider today's context for palliative care.

Leadership challenges in the current climate

The issues for health and social care at this point in history are huge, marked by the impact of the worldwide recession and significant demographic changes, with an increasingly elderly population and in comparison far less people of working age (certainly here in the UK). With the economic downturn cuts are continuing to bite. The UK National Health Service and Social Services Departments find themselves confronted with funding gaps demanding large-scale change. Of course the charitable sector is and will be equally affected. We live with ever closer scrutiny and accountability, resulting in much paperwork; we deal with an increasing complaint culture.

The leadership challenges in this context are equally huge, in terms of maintaining quality and productivity under tight budgets, in terms of continuing to deliver the best possible care and keeping the workforce engaged.

A key message from the National Health Service Institute for Innovation and Improvement in the UK is that in this climate organizations will only remain viable if able to focus at the level of the wider system as well as the organization. In other words, palliative care organizations will need to continue to look beyond the constraints of the 'hospice bubble', to step out from the inward-looking ways of the early pioneering days. They will need to focus at the organizational level and, crucially, to remain viable they will also need to continue to focus at the individual practitioner level. This takes us back to self-care and self-awareness. In tough times particularly, these can only be ignored at the organization's peril, tempting though it may be.

Leaders and their self-care

Clearly all of the above, how to practise relentless self-care and pursue rigorous self-awareness, applies to palliative care leaders as much as frontline workers. With the particular demands on leaders and the harsh context for health and social care overall, many will find themselves pedalling ever faster. And of course they will know about, at least intellectually, the importance of taking good care of themselves.

Leaders are likely to some degree to be driven, determined, and disciplined. Above I referred to the discipline required for relentless self-care. Let me put it to you that at times self-care can also be about the flip side, about breaking the discipline, stepping outside rules. David Oliviere, Director of Education and Training at St Christopher's Hospice, gives a lovely example of not returning to the office after the early finish of an event in town but instead enjoying a cappuccino and 'me time'. His delight in telling the story is infectious. On one level of course this is perfectly justifiable in terms of clawing back extra hours worked. On another level it does have the delicious feel of doing something ever so slightly delinquent.

Leaders may well be ambitious. This takes us back to the need for ordinariness. Leaders can feel disillusioned. This takes us back to the connection to purpose as part of self-care.

When demands crowd in, when the emails flood in ever faster, meetings get scheduled back to back and still there is that nurse or maybe social worker at your door, needing to bring to you a concern, maybe needing to speak some of the unspeakable in their work with the dying—can you still retain your ability to listen (and to take relevant action) whilst solidly, throughout, taking care of yourself? Or do you recognize a faint sinking feeling, perhaps panic rising or indeed numbness? Ultimately, I believe, taking care of ourselves in this context is about harnessing our capacity to stay connected with 'self', however pressurized we are.

Some may think of connectedness with self in terms of soul, that indefinable essence of a person's spirit and being. Soul cannot be touched and yet its absence can cause distress. In his exploration of the soul at work Whyte warns that sometimes 'work, paradoxically, does not ask enough of us, yet exhausts the narrow parts of us we do bring to its doors' (Whyte, 1997, p. 19). If, on the other hand, we are able to bring our soul into our work, remain connected with our self, then there is a chance of survival, and more.

Leaders and staff care

In relation to their workforce then leaders must take responsibility for both modelling their own self-care and facilitating their team's self-care. The latter, without a firm grounding in the former, will remain tokenistic and ultimately ineffective.

There is of course a broad range of potential vehicles for staff care, from more formal mechanisms such as team away days, peer-group or individual supervision, a team journal or open floor meetings, to informal team lunches and chats in the corridor. All of these are about shared conversations and shared reflection, with leaders holding the space and providing containment.

Here at St Christopher's Hospice in London the backbone of staff support is a clear framework for supervision, line management support, professional development, and a solid appraisal system. This structured approach is coupled with the maxim that managers, including the chief executive, will make themselves available when needed. Managers' doors are open. A culture of valuing and respecting all colleagues underpins the above, demonstrated in often seemingly small gestures. Avoiding overly sentimental initiatives (group hugs and lifesize teddy bears), it is nevertheless recognized that inevitably some patients will touch our hearts, sometimes deeply, and that at times we will find ourselves grieving for these patients. Allowing ourselves to experience grief and at other times keeping emotion at bay is considered healthy (thus ultimately avoiding grief overload, Papadatou, 2009, p. 159). Teams and individuals within teams have found various ways and rituals to mark and acknowledge deaths. Finally, occasional debriefing sessions are held for anybody immediately affected by particularly stressful or distressing events (such as a recent fatal road accident immediately outside the hospice).

Within this overall framework the individual leaders' style and approach to staff care will inevitably vary, based on their multiple experiences. My own is an eclectic one, influenced amongst much else by narrative therapy concepts, a collaborative model of supervision (Orlans and Edwards, 2001), personal lessons learnt from Scott Eberle's work (as described above), and many years of experience in palliative care. As their manager I am interested in building connections with team members, joining with their sense of what might be helpful to them at the time. From a stance of curiosity I will ask how I can support my team rather than assume that I know what is needed.

I will invite stories from individuals about how they experience themselves in their work, and explore with them how well these stories serve them and whether there may be alternative stories. I will enquire into stories of resilience in their work and seek out unspoken stories, always holding on to the notion of choice in what stories are told. It is worth remembering that stories can help and hinder. Arthur Frank writes compellingly about the trickster dangers of stories. 'Stories can trick us humans into understanding our lives in ways that impede and damage those lives' (Frank, 2009, p. 168). At times whole teams may hold onto powerful and potentially unhelpful stories about themselves, often reinforced by the wider organization, with new events interpreted to fit the script, new members coerced to follow the story line. This could be for instance the classic story of the underdogs who need to go to battle. In caring for the team I will go about unravelling and exploring some of those team stories, always in conversation with team members.

Rather than focusing on problems and difficulties I may use such conversations with team members also to discover *the best of what is* within the team and their particular work situation. Loosely based on the principles of Appreciative Enquiry (Cooperrider et al., 2008) the dialogue may move on to dreaming *what might be*, determining *what should be*, deciding *what will be*. This is a collaborative approach to staff support with a central co-created relationship between myself (the leader) and my team.

This relationship then becomes a supportive *container* for staff. The concept of the container goes back to the psychoanalyst Bion who likened it to the function of a mother whose ability to receive and process the overwhelming feelings of her baby makes these more bearable (Kearney, 2000, pp. 89, 90). In psychoanalytic therapy some of the work will be around tolerating feelings, previously projected onto others but gradually taken back, for long enough, in the safety of the containing relationship, so that change may become possible.

Linking mothers, babies, psychoanalysis, and staff support may seem far fetched. And yet, a similar process can become possible within a containing relationship between managers and their teams, not only in terms of individuals feeling safe enough to explore some difficult feelings but also in terms of them re-owning projections, for example taking back blame. This will go some way towards a reduction of polarization and antagonism amongst team members and promote integration and cooperation. This is staff care at its best.

Finally, much like Russian dolls, managers will be able to provide good containment if they are themselves contained. Throughout my own career I have found containment more than anything by actively seeking out mentors for myself, both formally and informally, in the shape of some (not all) line managers, some immediate colleagues, some peers in my wider professional network, and a supervisor.

Further reflections on leadership

Returning once more to the rigorous pursuit of self-awareness, that twin aspect of self-care, leaders in palliative care will need to reflect again and again on their leadership. What kind of leadership do they aspire to?

In a fascinating critical analysis of the key debates within leadership Western traces main leadership discourses as these have evolved from the early twentieth century (Western, 2008). 'Discourse' of course refers to the way society tends to think about certain topics (and in this case leadership), often representing what is out of consciousness. When identified though it becomes possible to step outside the discourse and reflect on our position in relation to it.

Of interest here is above all the 'Leader as Messiah' discourse, prominent from the 1970s and epitomized by the transformational 'hero' leader. These are leaders with charisma, who carry compelling visions in the face of an uncertain, turbulent environment. Their staff will work hard because of an internalized belief system aligned to their leaders' values. Many of the early pioneers in palliative care will have been such visionaries. Indeed the transformational hero leader discourse is still very much with us now (Lafferty, 1998; Barker, 2000).

As with all others, this leadership style has its merits as well as weak points. Western warns that leading from the Messiah position can be dangerous. Prophetic figures create disciples rather than active followers. At the same time such disciples will play their part in creating these visionary leaders as their collective unconscious fantasy seeks new hope in difficult times. Under such pressure it will take extraordinarily grounded leaders to stay firmly with their own ordinariness.

Interestingly, Western also identifies emergent new leadership thinking which he calls the Eco-leader discourse. 'Eco' here refers to interrelatedness. At the heart of this

discourse lies connectivity, looking beyond the closed system of individual organizations, focusing on networks, including stakeholders and the political and natural
environment. No longer can we survive in isolation. Eco-leadership does not try to
create strong cultures with homogeneous loyal employees, but the opposite, strong
networks which enable difference to flourish. As Western says: 'This discourse finds
that the real vulnerability of leadership lies in control, hierarchy and omnipotence.
The real strength of leadership lies in devolved power, dispersing leadership and
having the confidence of not-knowing' (Western, 2008, p. 197).

What Western terms the vulnerability in omnipotence relates to the dangerous
seductiveness of heroic dreams discussed above, be that for those with direct clinical
responsibility or indeed their leaders. Then, when Western writes of leadership
strength lying in having the confidence of not-knowing, this takes us to the ability to
tolerate incomplete understanding, termed 'negative capability' by the poet Keats
(1958), and in many ways the very antithesis to competence and decisive action so
often at the heart of traditional leadership. Alongside (not instead of) such positive
capabilities there may indeed be an argument for 'the capacity to sustain reflective
inaction' (Simpson et al., 2002, p. 1210), the leaders' capacity to see what is going on
in the moment, waiting in the place of uncertainty in order to allow for the emergence
of new thoughts and ideas.

Leadership from a *both*/*and* stance

Whatever leadership style we adopt, the key question still remains whether it is feasible
for leaders to do full justice to the demands of relentless self- and staff care whilst
delivering against targets and ensuring performance. Or, will these demands always sit
uncomfortably side by side, ultimately incompatible? Easy it certainly is not. The answer
I suggest lies in leadership from a *both*/*and* stance.

The following example should illustrate this stance. Some years ago I took responsibility for a redundancy, a decision driven by service development needs. Following traditional *either*/*or* thinking, I would have had to put to one side my considerations for the
welfare of the individual, albeit with some misgivings. However, from a *both*/*and* stance
I was able to *both* drive through necessary change *and* do this in the most humane way
possible. In very practical terms staff care here translated into my willingness to enter
into conversation despite the individual's anger and blame, not shirking responsibility,
giving transparent information. I expressed regret regarding the personal implications.
I did what I could to allow a dignified response. And, I paid attention to the impact on
the remaining team. Staff care here was not about protection from harsh realities.

Both/*and* leadership is also about holding *both* those positive capabilities *and* the negative capabilities discussed above, *both* clear direction *and* ambiguity. To give another
example, practitioners will frequently come to me with highly complex family scenarios
involving issues regarding safeguarding vulnerable individuals. Often decisions are
required here with regards to the duty to report to statutory services as well as strategies
for continued family work. These can be anxiety-provoking dilemmas requiring finely
tuned clinical judgement. What if we were to get it wrong? The temptation for me as the
leader may be to *take over* in an attempt to *take care*, by giving well-meant advice and
immediate guidance. From a both/and stance, however, I will often hold back, sit with

my own not-knowing, and allow answers to emerge in the dialogue. Taking care here is about *both* creating and holding space for conversation with the practitioner *and* at the same time indicating that I will share responsibility and ultimately be accountable for decisions taken.

Then, consider line-management supervision in terms of *both/and*. For practitioners to operate at their growing edge, managers will need to hold *both* a context where individual performance is scrutinized *and* a safe space where non-defensive awareness of areas of incompetence, vulnerability, and self-doubt is allowed, leading to greater competence and creative learning. Arguably this is a contradiction in terms. With both motivated, highly performing staff and those at the other end of the spectrum this tension between two different functions of line-management supervision is inevitable. Whilst sometimes uncomfortable, this calls for dialogue. Doing such groundwork around the relationship will pay off. Take for example the scenario of team members struggling with personal family issues that are affecting their work. In this scenario a solid relationship with the team members will be one crucial prerequisite allowing me to *both* show my care and offer support as a fellow human being and their manager, *and* to speak to them about their performance in a non-punitive and adult-to-adult manner.

Finally, when working with death, facing the uncontrollable and seemingly insurmountable, the pull for leaders to be in control and invulnerable is strong. Papadatou, however, echoing Winnicott's concept of the good-enough parent, challenges us to be vulnerable enough. Somewhere between being completely invulnerable and being highly vulnerable she suggests we find a place where 'when we are vulnerable enough, we are open and permeable to experiences and people' (Papadatou, 2009, p. 98). Can we let our teams see that we too wrestle with questions, doubts, and pressure?

It may seem there is a contradiction between containment, dependable relationships, and showing vulnerability. Once again this is about *both/and*. It is about being *both* solid *and* at the same time vulnerable enough. From that place connection with colleagues and staff support can follow.

Conclusion

The challenges of leadership in organizations delivering palliative care are multi-faceted, with leaders' self-care, self-awareness, and support for their teams underpinning the delivery of services. Most come to this field of work because of a particular interest or passion. Harnessing this engagement and nourishing continued resilience is not achieved by shielding ourselves and others from difficult realities nor with a stance of over-protectiveness. In contrast, we will continue to deliver 'good enough' services whilst taking care of ourselves and others if we are able to listen and stay present, rooted in our own competence and affirming others in theirs.

References

Barker, L. (2000). Effective leadership within hospice and palliative care units. *Journal of Management in Medicine*, **14**(5/6), 291–309.

Barnes, K. (2001). Staff stress in the children's hospice: Causes, effects and coping strategies. *International Journal of Palliative Nursing*, **7**(5), 248–54.

Cooperrider, D.L., Whitnet, D., and Stavros J.M. (2008). *Appreciative Enquiry Handbook: For Leaders of Change*. Brunswick: Crown Custom Publishing; San Francisco: Berrett-Koehler Publishers.

Eberle, S. (2006). *The Final Crossing: Learning to Die in Order to Live*. Big Pine, CA: Lost Borders Press.

Frank, A. (2009). The necessity and dangers of illness narratives, especially at the end of life. In Y. Gunaratnam and D. Oliviere (eds), *Narrative and Stories in Health Care: Illness, Dying and Bereavement*. Oxford: Oxford University Press.

Johnson, S.M. (1994). *Character Styles*. New York/London: W.W. Norton.

Katz, R.S. and Johnson, T.G. (eds) (2006). *When Professionals Weep: Emotional and Countertransference Responses in End-of-life Care*. London: Routledge.

Kearney, M. (1996). *Mortally Wounded: Stories of Soul Pain, Death and Healing*. Dublin: Marino Books.

Kearney, M. (2000). *A Place of Healing: Working with Suffering in Living and Dying*. Oxford: Oxford University Press.

Keats, J. (1958). Letter to George and Tom Keats, 21 December 1817. In H. E. Rollins (ed.), *The Letters of John Keats: 1814–1821*. Cambridge: Cambridge University Press.

Lafferty, C.L. (1998). Transformational leadership and the hospice R.N. case manager: A new critical pathway. *The Hospice Journal*, **13**(3), 35–48.

Monroe, B (2004). Emotional impact of palliative care on staff. In N. Sykes, P. Edmonds, and J. Wiles (eds), *Management of Advanced Disease*, 4th edn. London: Arnold.

Obholzer, A. and Roberts, V.Z. (eds) (1994). *The Unconscious at Work: Individual and Organizational Stress in the Human Services*. London: Routledge.

Orlans, V. and Edwards, D. (2001). A collaborative model of supervision. In M. Carroll and M. Tholstrup (eds), *Integrative Approaches to Supervision*. London: Jessica Kingsley.

Papadatou, D. (2009). *In the Face of Death: Professionals Who Care for the Dying and the Bereaved*. New York: Springer.

Payne, M. (2008). Staff support. In M. Lloyd-Williams (ed.), *Psychosocial Issues in Palliative Care*, 2nd edn. Oxford: Oxford University Press.

Renzenbrink, I. (2004). Relentless self care. In E.P. Silverman and J. Berzoff (eds), *Living with Dying: A Hand Book for Health Practitioners in End of Life Care*. New York: Columbia University Press.

Sherman, A.C. *et al.* (2006). Caregiver stress and burnout in an oncology unit. *Palliative and Supportive Care*, **4**(1), 65–80.

Simpson, P. and French, R. (2006). Negative capability and the capacity to think in the present moment: Some implications for leadership practice. *Leadership*, **2**(2), 245–55.

Simpson, P., French, R., and Harvey, C.E. (2002). Leadership and negative capability. *Human Relations*, **55**(10), 1209–26.

Vachon, M.L.S. (1995). Staff stress in hospice/palliative care: A review. *Palliative Medicine*, **9**, 91–122.

Western, S. (2008). *Leadership: A Critical Text*. London: Sage.

Whyte, D. (1997). *The Heart Aroused: Poetry and the Preservation of the Soul at Work*. London: Industrial Society.

Yalom, I.D. (2008). *Staring at the Sun: Overcoming the Dread of Death*. London: Piatkus.

Chapter 11

Seeing beyond the sadness: hope, resilience, and sustainable practice in childhood bereavement

Danny Nugus

Introduction

The principles and tools used in work with bereaved children offer meaningful insights for ensuring sustainable practice for workers in health and human services. Professionals ought not to feel sorry for clients, sad though their stories may be. Professionals serve their clients, themselves and their organizations better if they draw on and develop clients' resilience, potential, and hope. Similarly, professionals need resilience, supportive systems, and a balanced approach, rather than a spirit of self-sacrifice. This chapter will discuss the principles of childhood bereavement practice and apply them to professionals working in health and human services.

Certain traditional therapeutic principles hold that the expert professional 'gives' and the dependent client 'takes' (Brandon and Jack, 1997). In work with bereaved children, this translates to the professional taking on a responsibility for the grief and welfare of the child. Professionals who feel responsible for clients' problems become overwhelmed and cannot sustain practice in the long term (Renzenbrink, 2004; Dolan and Nelson, 2007). This dichotomy of 'giving' and 'taking' suggests a trade-off between looking after oneself (by doing less) or giving more to help the client at one's own expense; and a belief that good outcomes require enormous (and unsustainable) outputs of emotional and physical energy. Failure of individuals and organizations to build the capacity of professionals makes them, and their organizations, susceptible to burnout, illness, and compassion fatigue (Stebnicki, 2007; Worden, 2009).

Contemporary bereavement practice, with specific reference to solution-focused approaches, centres increasingly on the resources, responsibility, and expertise of clients (e.g. Simon, 2010; de Castro and Guterman, 2008; Butler and Powers, 1996; Gray, Zide, and Wilker, 2000; Nugus, 2009). Solution-focused brief therapy (SFBT) was pioneered by Steve de Shazer, Insoo Kim Berg, and colleagues at the Milwaukee Family Therapy Center, USA, in the early to mid 1980s (de Shazer, 1985, 1988; de Shazer and Dolan, 2007; Cade, 2007). SFBT invites a focus on what is possible rather than what is not: on strengths and resources, not weaknesses and deficits; on people, not problems; on cooperation, not resistance; on movement, not 'stuck-ness'; and on doing more of what is working and less of what is not. This enables a person to take small achievable steps towards the life they want to be leading (e.g. Iveson, in McKergow and Glass, 2010; Berg and Steiner, 2003; Selekman, 1997; Burns, 2005; Nelson, 2010). Such an approach offers clarity, control, and confidence to move forward in the presence of grief and other problems. The imperative of an empowering approach in childhood bereavement and, more broadly, health and human services is also supported by an abundance of research in other areas of healthcare (e.g. Moseley, 2004; Harrow et al., 2009; Moos and Moos, 2007; Vauth et al., 2007). Facilitating understanding that grief is a normal and necessary response to death and loss, and helping clients and professionals to maximize and build their resources, enables positive and sustainable outcomes for clients and professionals alike.

This chapter considers four principles of childhood bereavement practice. These principles have been developed over 20 years' experience in the field of childhood bereavement and also draw upon the tradition and practice of SFBT. These principles inform and are informed by the work of Winston's Wish, the charity for bereaved children in the United Kingdom. The first principle is recognizing and *building the capacity* of clients. The second principle is *enabling control* for the client. The third principle is that professionals should recall that *it is the client's grief* and, therefore, not for professionals to try and remove or resolve grief. The fourth principle concerns helping clients to accept *grief as normal and necessary*. Health and human service organizations and professionals must also enact these principles, so that capacity and control are developed for sustainable practice.

Promoting the independence of clients leads to a more sustainable and effective way of working. I discuss this in relation to each of the four principles. Many ways to help children who are bereaved that will be discussed in this chapter apply also to bereaved adults. However, the concept of bereavement in children invokes particular anxiety (Dyregrov, 2008). This makes the lessons they offer particularly potent for professionals' and organizations' sustainability. Staff working in health and human services ought to apply the principles of: building capacity; enabling control; placing responsibility for needs on clients rather than themselves; and recognizing that challenges and difficulties are normal aspects of work life.

Building capacity

When professionals at Winston's Wish see a child who has been bereaved, we strive to see a child with potential and strength, rather than an object of pity. People who are bereaved can learn to 'grow around their grief'. They need to be able to become resilient and resourceful adults. Resilience can be understood as 'a dynamic process encompassing positive adaptation within the context of significant adversity' (Luthar et al., in Salloum and Rynearson, 2006, p. 50). This idea of adapting and building capacity is captured in a model by Tonkin (1996) called 'Growing Around Grief '(Figure 11.1).

The model represents an understanding of how people grieve and adjust to life following the death of someone important. Each bottle (A, B, C, D) represents the grieving person's life and capacity. The ball represents grief and all the pain, despair, changes, additional losses, and difficulties associated with it.

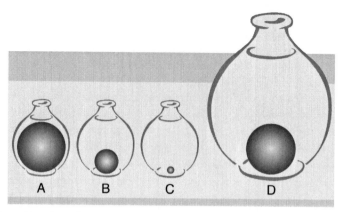

Fig. 11.1 Tonkin's (1996) 'Growing Around Grief' model.

In bottle 'A', the ball of grief fills the whole bottle—a normal response for a bereaved person. Bottles 'B' and 'C' represent traditional theories of bereavement, suggesting that, through a 'grief work approach', the grief gets smaller over time, culminating in resolution and recovery (critiqued by Wortman and Silver, 1989, and Bonanno, 1999). Similarly, challenging conventional bereavement theories, bottle 'D' suggests that one's grief does not merely diminish with the passing of time. The ball remains the same size in bottle 'D'. The depiction of grief in bottle 'D' validates the intensity and pervasiveness of grief, rather than minimizing it. It represents one's capacity to 'grow around grief', incorporating it into one's future. The bereaved person accommodates, adapts, lives with, and may even grow from, their grief.

This model works when applied to children because it normalizes and validates a child's grief. Children who are bereaved do not necessarily want to remove the grief. Often relationships with the deceased are tied to the way children grieve and are important for living with the grief in the future. As one of our service users explained:

> In some ways the pain of grief itself stayed much the same . . . But as time went on my world expanded so it felt less suffocating.

'Stephen', 16, was 10 when his mother died. He and his family attended a Winston's Wish residential group for families bereaved by suicide. He offered the following reflection with his peers and group facilitators when the 'Growing Around Grief' model was shared:

> For me it's like a barbed-wire fence. But a hedge has grown around it. That's me just trying to live with it. I'm trying to get on with life. But the fence is always there, even if other people can't see it. It still hurts and catches me sometimes but it's not the only thing that's in my life now. Remembering Mum—who she was—and knowing that it's not just me . . . it's like the hedge is starting to bloom.

In essence, capacity for living with grief has been held to involve a number of inter-related features. These include: strong social support networks; the presence of at least one unconditionally supportive parent or parent substitute; positive school experiences;

a sense of mastery and a belief that one's own efforts can make a difference; participation in events outside school and the home; the capacity to reframe adversities so that the beneficial effects are recognized; the ability, or the recognition, to make a difference by helping others or through part-time work (for teenagers); and not to be excessively sheltered from challenging situations which provide opportunities to develop coping skills (Newman, 2003; Stubbs et al., 2006; Bonanno, 2008).

Health and human service professionals also need to build their capacity. What bereaved children require for building capacity offers valuable meaning and guidance for becoming, or remaining, robust and dependable professionals. The child's family relationships and how they adjust and move forward in a way that works for them is what matters most, not their therapeutic 'relationship' with us or what we can do for them. The client, rather than the professional, needs to be the central decision-maker in the support that they receive. This is a more sustainable and empowering way of working because it preserves the resources of professionals and expands the client's resources.

Empowering, collaborative, and non-paternalistic childhood bereavement practices involve working in ways that draw out and draw upon a child or young person's own capabilities, resources, and support networks. This requires a propensity to trust in the client's capacity to change (Rogers, 1951). Winston's Wish offers a family-focused approach and facilitates opportunities for children to meet others their age who are similarly bereaved. The aim is to see these efforts and interventions complementing, not replicating or replacing, what is already being done well to help children and their families navigate their way through grief (Nugus and Stokes, 2007). This enables sustainable working because it shares responsibility, empowers service users, and mobilizes their supporters.

The 'Growing Around Grief' model is invariably greeted with nodding heads when shared with other professionals in training contexts. My colleagues and I have successfully applied this model to assist professionals in identifying resources and strategies to manage the emotional demands of working with children who have been bereaved. It has also been beneficial in helping health and human service professionals to increase their emotional threshold to be able to listen to children's stories.

In Figure 11.1, the depiction of the ball remaining the same size (A and D) validates the challenges of grief and loss for professionals and normalizes their anxieties. The 'growing' metaphor invites health and human service professionals to consider what they are already doing and can do more of to create space in their professional and personal lives for other things—to achieve balance so that the work does not become suffocating or begin to 'spill out of the bottle'. This conceptualization focuses on solutions and ways for professionals to move forward and restore hope for themselves and their clients in the presence of grief and ongoing difficulties (Nugus, 2009; Simon, 2010; Hackett, 2008; Fiske, 2008; Dolan and Nelson, 2007).

Sometimes adults, including professionals, avoid addressing grief on the terms set by children who are bereaved. When training and speaking with colleagues in the children's workforce about childhood bereavement I invariably hear comments such as: 'I don't want to say the wrong thing', 'I'm not qualified', 'I'm worried I'll get upset', and 'I might make it worse'. In fact it is unlikely that what we say or do will make matters worse (Dyregrov, 2008). The greater risk is that non-action, stifled initiative, and an inability to talk directly and honestly about death will leave a bereaved child feeling more vulnerable, disempowered, and isolated than they already are.

Professionals who avoid addressing grief directly might think they are being helpful and protective. However, these well-intentioned comments arguably represent a focus on the fear, anxieties, and protection of the professional, rather than the needs of the client (Dyregrov, 2008; Finegan and McGurk, 2007; Newburger and Bourne, 1985; Silverman, 2000). Confronting and addressing grief on the terms defined by the client can enable professionals to build their own capacity, in parallel with that of their clients. This can build skills and confidence to provide a meaningful response in difficult areas of work.

Enabling control

Children who are bereaved need to know that they can shape their future and they can have some control and influence over what is happening within and around them. Following the death of someone important, children experience tremendous emotional and environmental upheaval. Bereavement heightens anxieties, confusion, and enforced changes beyond a child's control—and through no choice or fault of their own. Therefore, professionals and other adults need to inform children and offer choices to give them back some power and control. The client rather than the professional ought to be the centre of the model of support.

Children who are bereaved can be empowered through involvement in rituals such as the funeral ceremony. They can also be given choice over the ways in which they remember the person who died, be given information in language they understand and a confident story about the death that they can tell others if they choose to. This is how a child can begin to increase their control over their grief and their future rather than be dependent on bereavement professionals and support organizations.

Children derive control from grieving in their own unique ways. There is no right or wrong way to grieve (Stokes, 2004; Salloum and Rynearson, 2006; de Castro and Guterman, 2008; Nugus and Stokes, 2007) and it is a complex and personal process. Services and support should therefore strive to be non-prescriptive, individualized, flexible, relevant to children, client-led, and designed to support children in the context of their family and existing support systems (Nugus and Stokes, 2007). Respecting, listening to, and learning from children as individuals need to be the foundations of supporting children who have been bereaved. For professionals, this relieves the pressure to try and have all the answers or remedies, and thus lends itself to working sustainably.

Selekman (1997) suggests that when working with traumatized children,

> we need to empower them to become masters of their own lives . . . by conveying an optimistic attitude, capitalizing on their competency areas (and what is 'going right' in their present lives), respecting their defenses, and giving them room to tell their painful stories when, and if, they choose to do so.

Children who are bereaved will express to others the character of their grief, and how they want their lives to be, if given appropriate opportunities. Children's bereavement work must involve 'one foot in pain and one foot in possibility' (O'Hanlon, 2003; Rees, 2008), so that they can focus on and feel more in control of their past, present, and future.

The extent of one's sense of control has significant implications for children and for the way that professionals approach work with them. Schuurman (2003) associates higher levels of anxiety, depression, pessimism, health problems, under-performance, and lower self-esteem in bereaved children with them having an *external* locus of control—that is the belief that one's fate is in someone else's hands. It has also been shown that childhood bereavement is associated with comparatively poorer outcomes in health, education, social, and personal indicators for bereaved children than their peers (Greene et al., 2004; Fauth et al., 2009).

The need for a child who is bereaved to be more in control of their past, present, and future in order to improve their outcomes is also mirrored by an abundance of research in other areas of medicine and healthcare—for example in the fields of chronic pain (e.g. Rosenfeld et al., 2003; Moseley, 2004) and psychology (e.g. Harrow et al., 2009; Bandura, 1997). In further support of the principles underpinning this chapter, the research across these fields powerfully demonstrates that a greater sense of control and influence, strong self-efficacy and an adaptive capacity are essential for managing difficulties and sustaining that which is helpful.

Five particular traits or predispositions are identified as being important to developing resilience (part of what I am calling 'capacity') in children who are bereaved. These are the need for: an *internal* locus of control; healthy self-esteem; easy-going temperament; affection; and well-developed reasoning skills (Schuurman, 2003). As professionals we can reflect on which of these can, or need to, be identified and nurtured in ourselves to develop our capacity, alongside supporting clients to develop theirs.

The sustainability of practice in childhood bereavement work depends on professionals being able to approach their work from a collaborative position that stems from normalizing grief, rather than 'caring for', 'helping', or trying to 'fix' or pathologize grief. This perspective challenges a traditional dichotomy between 'professional giving' and 'client receiving'. Enabling control for the client also enables control, clearer definition of roles and boundaries, and self-preservation and sustainable practice for professionals in health and human services.

To genuinely shift the balance of control back towards the child, professionals need to employ methods and communicate in ways that are accessible for the child. Metaphors and creative activities can be powerful and flexible tools. They can enable children who are bereaved to conceptualize their grief adaptively, and have hope for the future in the presence of grief (Stubbs, Nugus, and Gardner, 2008; Stokes, 2004). Children need to be able to explore, express, and manage their grief in unique ways that promote choice, control, and a focus on the future. This helps to foster a 'resilient mind-set' (Stokes, 2004) and a focus on living well, not just coping. Therefore, clients feel more empowered and professionals' capacity for working with clients is preserved and energized.

Winston's Wish practitioners use a 'film strip' story technique, described by McIntyre and Hogwood (2006), to help enable a child to 'take control' of their story.

The children we support often report that particular intrusive images and sensory stimuli play 'on loop' in their heads. The metaphor of a film reel invites children to 'eject', through drawing, writing, or both, onto the film-reel paper, their personal sequential story of what happened when the person died, incorporating a beginning, a middle, and an ending. Once completed and having shared it if they choose to, the children are invited to keep it somewhere safe. They are reminded that they can now choose when they want to 'rent it out' or 'press play'. This gives control over the role of their memories and thoughts.

A recent, typical response came from 'Dylan', now 12, who was 9 when he witnessed his father murder his mother. He engaged in the film-reel activity facilitated in a small group with other boys and girls his age, similarly bereaved through murder or manslaughter. He told us three months later:

> When I think of Mum now I mostly remember the good times, more than what happened [when she died]. And I've started playing football again.

A teenage girl who survived a road traffic accident, in which her mother and younger brother died, explained the benefit of similar support using the metaphor of her computer, a lifeline for her to access online support:

> It [the memory of the car accident] is still on my hard-drive, but no longer on my desk-top. I try not to download it, only when I want to think about it.

Similarly, professionals need opportunities to externalize difficult stories and experiences. We should not try to be 'super-professionals'. We must consider and share the impact that events at work and elsewhere have on us, in light of the emotional demands of our work and our own individual circumstances. We need to be able to express our 'stories' and process them adaptively with the support of trusted peers. We need to be able to sleep well and limit the potential for our work lives to impact negatively on our home and personal lives, and vice versa. By being in control of our own stories, we are more likely to be able to support people in a manner that leaves our inbuilt prejudices, assumptions, and personal needs and anxieties to one side, and balance a lightness of touch with confidence and pragmatism. To be able to sustainably work with clients who are bereaved or seriously ill, professionals need an organizational culture and leadership that recognizes and prioritizes such support (Renzenbrink, 2004; Dyregrov, 2008). As professionals who support bereaved children, we need not only work towards increasing a child or young person's level of control in their own lives and futures. We should also consider how we can better understand and exercise control for ourselves and our practice, on a personal level. In the tradition of being solution focused, professionals would do well to 'identify what's working and do more of it' (de Jong and Berg, 2001; Macdonald, 2007; Dolan and Nelson, 2007). To develop sustainable work practices one needs to learn from and apply to oneself what children have reported to be beneficial and what we understand to be contributing factors in promoting resilience and nurturing hope (Fiske, 2008) in the lives of bereaved children.

As Baruch Shalum puts it, 'There is nothing wrong with you that what is right with you couldn't fix' (cited in O'Connell, 1998, p. 19).

It's their grief not ours

Professionals dealing with children who are bereaved need to recall that it is the child's grief, not theirs. Children who are bereaved are the experts in their own lives and what their grief means to them. Professionals cannot presume to know everything that is best for a child in their life. Equally, professionals ought not to take responsibility for the child's grief. Solution-focused brief therapists, for example, are guided by the principle to not work harder than the client (Macdonald, 2007). We need to ask them what they wish for themselves, ask them to consider what living well—not just 'coping'—means to them, and be curious about what they already do, or have previously done, that helps. This can help to amplify the child's capacity to employ resources, strategies, and meaning that help them now and into the future.

Supporting the child in the context of his or her family, providing opportunities for facilitated peer support, and mobilizing the existing support around the child (e.g. school) help to share responsibility whilst keeping the individual child central and empowered (Stokes, 2004; Nugus and Stokes, 2007; Selekman, 1997). In health and human services generally, carrying the burden of responsibility for clients' outcomes is detrimental for well-intentioned professionals and the clients themselves. Such approaches are misguided and less effective because they are unsustainable for both client and professional. They fail to utilize and give credit to the client as the primary resource in realizing their 'preferred future' (George, Iveson, and Ratner, 1999).

Professional guidance needs to develop the client's resources to be independent of the professional (Kelly, 2010). This does not mean withdrawing support or compromising empathy. Instead it supports the child to draw on their own internal and external resources in order to make sense of their bereavement and learn to live with their grief. If we as professionals are disturbed by children's grief, we need to process that elsewhere. We need to deal with children in a non-shocked, non-judgemental, non-'sympathetic', non-patronizing, non-amateurish, and professional manner, aligning self-awareness with emotional attunement. My colleague, Brendan McIntyre, describes this awareness and ability to engage with a child and have normal, and therapeutically useful, conversations about death and dying as 'sophisticated ordinariness'.

For a child who is bereaved to achieve his or her desired outcome requires them to have ownership of the meaning-making process (Niemeyer, 2001). If we perceive children to have the capacity for resilience even when presently vulnerable, we will be less likely to withhold information from them or do things for them (or to them), rather than with them. We will be more likely to lead from one step behind (Cantwell and Holmes, 1994) and work creatively and in a child-friendly way (Berg and Steiner, 2003). The alternative is to direct or be rigid, scripted or avoidant, all of which would render our efforts less effective, less relevant, and less accessible for the child we are endeavouring to help.

As with *enabling control*, the principle that *it's their grief, not ours* can be applied as an organizational perspective. The objectives of care, end-of-life, and bereavement work must be relevant and meaningful for the professional in the context of the needs of the organization. The professional must be at the centre of all decisions relating to how to develop professionally. To retain, sustain, and support staff within a culture of trust and appreciation, the management style and structure and organization need to embody the values that underpin the work we strive to do.

Normal and necessary

Bereavement is not an illness, despite advocacy for its inclusion in the fifth edition of the Diagnostic and Statistical Manual of Mental Disorders (DSM-V) (Lichtenthal, Cruess, and Prigerson, 2004; critiqued in Aldhous, 2009). Grief is a normal and natural response to one of the most painful and isolating experiences a child can ever face (Nugus and Stokes, 2007; Nugus, 2009). Children and adults who are bereaved oscillate between preoccupation with grief and the deceased (loss orientation), and managing daily activities (restoration orientation), such as putting on the school uniform to go to school. This normal, dynamic, and functional response is known as the dual-process model for coping with bereavement (Stroebe and Schut, 1999). The emotions associated with grief are a normal and necessary part of grieving and living with grief.

For instance, when my Winston's Wish colleagues and I meet children and their families, we never say 'I'm sorry about your loss'. The greeting is more likely to proceed as follows: 'Really nice to meet you', 'Good to put a face to the voice', 'How's your morning been?', 'What's your cat's name?' (if when we visit them at home we see a pet cat), and so on. The normality of grief involves maintaining a connection with the person who has died, rather than severing attachment at the time of death. This understanding relates to the theory of continuing bonds (Klass, Silverman, and Nickman, 1996). Children who are bereaved need to find an appropriate place for the person who has died in the context of their ongoing lives (Stokes, 2004).

Emotions associated with grief are normal and necessary. Children who are bereaved need to engage in a meaning-making process (Niemeyer, 2001). This involves a child interpreting, expressing, and internalizing what the death experience means to them. In order to do this, children who are bereaved need information about the death. This helps them to work out 'how' and 'why' the person died and also what role this person can now have in their lives.

The importance of living a balanced life reflects the normality of grief. To achieve and maintain a balanced life, develop a positive self-identity and feel in control following the death of a parent, Brewer (2009) recommends a 'moving-wheel model of living with bereavement' (Figure 11.2). This model emphasizes the need for children who are bereaved to maintain the following elements in their lives: physical activity; expressing emotion; positive adult relationships; strengthening areas of competence; developing and enhancing friendships; social support; and having fun and sharing humour.

A strong emphasis of Brewer's model is supportive networks, such as the family. These elements form a balance among the spokes in the life of a bereaved child, to enable movement oiled by a healthy self-identity and a sense of control over the future which children need. It may seem counter-intuitive to consider humour as a potentially useful tool in grieving, both for the child who is bereaved and the professional. However, we should not assume that humour is 'off limits', although it should be used with discretion. Humour, like grief, is normal and necessary. It can be disarming,

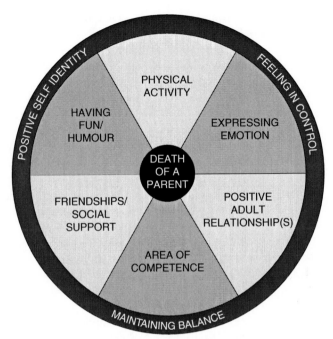

Fig. 11.2 Moving-wheel model of living with bereavement (Brewer, 2009).

stress-relieving, a good 'leveller' to offset the professional–client power imbalance, and may be the shortest distance between two people. It can be a vital coping mechanism and a conduit for the re-emergence of normality, optimism, and future happiness in the face of adversity and sadness (Horowitz, 2009; Bonanno, 1999; Brewer 2009; Vanistendael, 2008; Gajos, 2003). Humour may therefore be a vital ingredient also needed by professionals for a balanced life, a healthy workplace, and sustainable practice.

Given that grief is a normal experience, Brewer's model reminds professionals of the need to have the whole child in mind, not just their bereavement, when offering them bereavement support. This will help the child to broaden their own worldview, consider possibilities, and recognize their own internal and external resources and coping mechanisms. This can empower a bereaved child and represents a less intensive and therefore more sustainable way of working for the professional. Furthermore, the model draws attention to the need for professionals to live a balanced, self-nurturing life, to be able to continue to work in health and human services.

Sustainability: what works in practice?

Vehicles of expression, such as those outlined above, can reinforce affirming messages that normalize difficult experiences and give permission for self-care. This is true for professionals as it is for children who are bereaved. Similarly, creative therapeutic tools that are used with children can also enable a professional to identify, activate, and utilize their external and internal resources and support mechanisms. Indeed, use of stimuli such as metaphors, literature, and resourceful activities invites professionals to consider their own well-being as well as the client's. Implicit in this is the need for self-care and self-awareness among professionals, not self-sacrifice. Working with clients in empowering and collaborative ways can sustain our practice whilst helping to sustain those whom we endeavour to support.

Professionals can learn a lot from bereaved children. The 'dual-process model' should apply equally to staff as to children who are bereaved. Professionals also need to identify how they want their lives to be and use strategies that impact positively on their own future. Ongoing support strategies and peer support mechanisms can optimize staff performance through coping efficacy (Dowdall-Thomae et al., 2009). Like continuing bonds, relationships need to be nurtured and prioritized to allow staff to debrief, especially in the context of external work pressures and stressors.

My colleagues and I benefit from working in pairs ('co-working'). This allows a shared responsibility, close and non-competitive working relationships, affirmation of skills and abilities, opportunities to learn and develop, and organic opportunities for peer support, in addition to our formal structures (e.g. monthly peer supervision meetings peer case management meetings, and external supervision paid for by our employer). It also enables flexibility, choice, and greater accessibility for service users. We consider that quality control and staff support can and should go hand-in-hand.

If grief itself is an individual journey, so too are professional journeys. Each professional needs different levels and different types of support, and for different reasons. These needs will evolve and change depending on what is occurring for individual team members at any given time in their own lives. An open recognition of and responsiveness to the influence of individual issues and pressures can give permission for self-care without inference. These issues may include our own bereavements and losses, relationship difficulties, pregnancy and parenthood, illness, workload, and external commitments. This approach to self-care must become part of the fabric of a healthy organization. Indeed, the management style, structure, and organizational ethos need to embody the values that underpin the work we do.

Professional support structures, such as those discussed above, will help organizations to match the suitability of professionals to the organization and to particular roles or tasks. They also provide a framework for sustainability and job satisfaction. Staff whose motivations, interests, and aspirations match those of the organization are more likely to report satisfaction at work (Locke and Latham, 1990). Recruitment, induction, and performance appraisal processes ought to identify the particular needs, experiences, aspirations, expectations, interests, and motivations of staff. Each professional should be heavily involved in the design of their own performance appraisal and development programme, which should be flexible enough to adapt over time to meet changing needs of the professional, clients, and organization. The shared organizational, peer, and individual responsibilities for ensuring sustainable practice are even more pertinent in a pressured financial and political climate where there is an increasing need and expectation to 'do more with less'.

Many health and human service professionals extol the virtues of self-care to clients and colleagues. Professionals and organizations must 'practise what we preach' to make our work sustainable. This involves open communication, promoting choice and control, and focusing on the future development of the workforce and staffing profile. Organizations must facilitate reflexive engagement among professionals. A reflective organization facilitates the critical discussion among staff at various levels of clinical and organizational practices. Organizational reflexivity involves critical and communal reflection on practice, which might stimulate practice change. Such practices might inspire confidence among professionals to acknowledge limitations, and address concerns, grievances, and pressures before they become unmanageable. The alternative is a competition in which staff seek to outperform each other as 'super-clinicians'. Reflective organizations have more capacity to absorb the impact of stories and the inevitable impact of the emotionally challenging work of health and human services in professionals' work lives.

Conclusion

Children who have been bereaved have capabilities to do great things and 'live the lives they richly deserve' (Wheeler, 2008), even in the face of extreme adversity and profound loss. They have resources within them and around them that they are using, even if they do not yet know it, perhaps just to get through the day. Enabling ownership, facilitating understanding that grief is normal and necessary, and building capacity and control develops resources and sustainability for clients and professionals, and organizations who serve them both.

When working with people who are bereaved, we need to be mindful that it is their grief and not our role to take it away. We can build trust and confidence and convey empathy without letting sympathy and sadness become the all-pervading and disabling narrative or context for the work we do together. Thus, professionals can remove the burden of responsibility for the problem and the solution which can be a stressor for professionals working with children where the emotional content and desire to make a difference is high. Through applying these principles to practice, both professional and client can see beyond the sadness to ensure meaningful, lasting outcomes that are more sustainable, for the child because they own them, and for the worker, because they do not.

Many of the principles discussed in this chapter relate to bereavement work generally. However, working with children evokes particular anxiety among professionals and adults. This means that principles with which to support children who are bereaved ought to have particular resonance for the preservation of professionals. Those working on the frontlines in the field of childhood bereavement, and in other health and human service organizations, are prone to emotional stress and in need of support to practise sustainably. Children can grow from their grief. Seeing beyond the sadness can equally help to nourish, motivate, and inspire professionals to grow with and from the demanding but richly rewarding work we do.

References

Alilovic, K. (2004). Beyond the rough rock: Offering a specialist group for families bereaved by suicide. In J. Stokes (ed.), *Then, Now and Always: Supporting Children as they Journey Through Grief: A Guide for Practitioners*. Cheltenham: Winston's Wish, 155–77.

Bandura, A. (1997). *Self-efficacy: The Exercise of Control*. New York: Freeman.

Berg, I.K. and Steiner, T. (2003). *Children's Solution Work*. New York: Norton.

Bonanno, G.A. (1999). Emotional dissociation, self-deception, and adaptation to loss. In C.R. Figley (ed.), *Traumatology of Grieving: Conceptual, Theoretical, and Treatment Foundations*. Philadelphia: Brunner/Mazel, 89–108.

Bonanno, G.A. (2008). Loss, trauma, and human resilience: Have we underestimated the human capacity to thrive after extremely aversive events? *Psychological Trauma: Theory, Research, Practice, and Policy*, **S**(1), 101–13.

Brandon, D. and Jack, R. (1997). Struggling with services. In I.J. Norman and S.J. Redfern (eds), *Mental Health Care for Elderly People*. Norfolk, UK: Churchill Livingstone.

Brewer, J. (2009). Living with bereavement: An ethnographic study of young people's experiences of parental death. Doctoral dissertation, School of Sport and Health Sciences, University of Exeter, UK.

Burns, K. (2005). *Focus on Solutions: A Health Professional's Guide*. London: Whurr.

Butler, W.R. and Powers, K.V. (1996) Solution-focused grief therapy. In S.D. Miller, M.A. Hubble, and B.L. Duncan (eds), *Handbook of Solution-focused Brief Therapy*. San Francisco: Jossey-Bass, 228–47.

Cade, B. (2007). Springs, streams and tributaries: A history of the brief, solution-focused approach. In T.S. Nelson and F.N. Thomas (eds), *Handbook of Solution Focused Brief Therapy: Clinical Applications*. Philadelphia: Hawthorn Press, 25–64.

Cantwell, P. and Holmes, S.S. (1994). Social construction: A paradigm shift for systemic therapy and training. *The Australian and New Zealand Journal of Family Therapy*, **15**, 17–26.

de Castro, S. and Guterman, J.T. (2008). Solution-focused therapy for families coping with suicide. *Journal of Marital and Family Therapy*, **34**(1), 93–106.

deJong, P. and Berg, I.K. (2001). *Interviewing for Solutions*. London: Wadsworth.

deShazer, S. (1985). *Keys to Solution in Brief Therapy*. New York: Norton.

deShazer (1988). *Clues: Investigating Solutions in Brief Therapy*. New York: Norton.

deShazer, S. and Dolan, Y. (2007). *More than Miracles: The State of the Art of Solution Focused Brief Therapy*. New York: Haworth.

Dolan, Y. and Nelson, T. (2007). 'This job is so demanding': Using solution-focused questions to assess and relieve burnout. In T.S. Nelson and F.N. Thomas (eds), *Handbook of Solution Focused Brief Therapy: Clinical Applications*. Philadelphia, PA: Hawthorn Press, 249–66.

Dowdall-Thomae, C., Culliney, S., and Piechura, J. (2009). Peer support action plan: Northwest fire and rescue (Tucson, Arizona). *International Journal of Emergency Mental Health*, **11**(3), 177–83.

Duncan, B.L., Miller, S.D., and Sparks, J.A. (2003). Interactional and solution-focused brief therapies: Evolving concepts of change. In T.L. Sexton, G.R. Weeks, and T.S. Robbins (eds), *Handbook of Family Therapy*. New York: Brunner-Routledge, 101–23.

Dyregrov, A. (2008). *Grief In Children: A Handbook for Adults*, 2nd edn. London: Jessica Kingsley.

Finegan, W.C. and McGurk, A. (2007). *Care of the Cancer Patient: A Quick Reference Guide*. Oxford: Radcliffe.

Fiske, H. (2008). *Hope in Action: Solution Focused Conversations About Suicide*. Philadelphia: Hawthorn Press.

Gajos, E.M. (2003). *Regaining a Healthy Lifestyle after Bereavement—The Therapeutic Use of Humour in Counselling Therapy*. Sheffield: Sheffield Hallam University. Annales Universitatis Mariae Curie-Sklodowska, Lublin, Polonia, **58**(13), 303 (D).

George, E., Iveson, C., and Ratner, H. (1999). *Problem to Solution: Brief Therapy with Individuals and Families*. London: BT Press.

Gingerich, W. and Eisengart, S. (2000). Solution-focused brief therapy: A review of the outcome research. *Family Process*, **39**, 477–98.

Gray, S., Zide, M.R., and Wilker, H. (2000). Using the solution focused brief therapy model with bereavement groups in rural communities: Resiliency at its best. *The Hospice Journal* (now *Journal of Pain and Palliative Care Pharmacotherapy*), **15**(3): 13–30.

Greene, G.J., Lee, M.-Y., Trask, R., and Rheinscheld, J. (2005). How to work with clients' strengths in crisis intervention: A solution-focused approach. In A.R. Roberts (ed.), *Crisis Intervention Handbook: Assessment, Treatment and Research*, 3rd edn. Oxford: Oxford University Press, 64–89.

Hackett, P. (2008). How do solution focused practitioners deal with grief and grieving? MSc dissertation, Family and Systemic Psychotherapy, Birkbeck College, University of London, in collaboration with Institute of Family Therapy.

Harrow, M., Hansford, B.G., and Astrachan-Fletcher, E.B. (2009). Locus of control: Relation to schizophrenia, to recovery, and to depression and psychosis—A 15-year longitudinal study. *Psychiatry Research*, **168**(3), 186–92.

Henden, J. (2008). *Preventing Suicide: The Solution Focused Approach*. Chichester: Wiley.

Horowitz, S. (2009). Effect of positive emotions on health: Hope and humor. *Alternative and Complementary Therapies*, **15**(4), 196–202.

Kelly, A. (2010). *With Head, Heart and Hand: Dimensions of Community Building*, 2nd edn. Brisbane: Boolarong Press.

Klass, D., Silverman, P.R., and Nickman, S. (1996). *Continuing Bonds: New Understandings of Grief*. Washington DC: Taylor and Francis.

Lefcourt, F.M. (2001). The humor solution. In C.R. Snyder(ed.), *Coping With Stress: Effective People and Processes*. New York: Oxford University Press, 68–92.

Lichtenthal, W.G., Cruess, D.G., and Prigerson, H.G. (2004). A case for establishing complicated grief as a distinct mental disorder in DSM-V. *Clinical Psychology Review*, **24**(6), 637–62.

Locke, E.A. and Latham, G.P. (1990). Work motivation and satisfaction: Light at the end of the tunnel. *Psychological Science*, **1**, 240–6.

Macdonald, A. (2007). *Solution-focused Therapy: Theory, Research and Practice*. London: Sage.

McKergow, M. and Glass, C. (2010). Chris Iveson: Striving towards minimalism in changing scenery (interview). *InterAction*, **2**(1), 122–32.

McIntyre, B. and Hogwood, J. (2006). Play, stop and eject: Creating film strip stories with bereaved young people. *Bereavement Care*, **25**, 3.

Moos, R.H. and Moos, B.S. (2007). Protective resources and long-term recovery from alcohol use disorders. *Drug and Alcohol Dependence*, **86**(1), 46–54.

Moseley, G.L. (2004). Evidence for a direct relationship between cognitive and physical change during an education intervention in people with chronic low back pain. *European Journal of Pain*, **8**(1), 39–45.

Niemeyer, R.A. (ed.) (2001). *Meaning Reconstruction and the Experience of Loss*. Washington DC: American Psychological Association.

Nelson, T. (ed.) (2010). *Doing Something Different: Solution Focused Brief Therapy Practices*. New York: Routledge.

Newberger, E.H. and Bourne, R. (1985). *Unhappy Families: Clinical and Research Perspectives on Family Violence*. Oxford: Mosby.

Newman, T. (2003). *Promoting Resilience: A Review of Effective Strategies for Child Care Services.* University of Exeter, UK: Centre for Evidence Based Social Services.

Nugus, D. (2009). Choosing life: Solution focused approaches with suicide-bereaved young people who self-harm. *Counselling Children and Young People*, March, 32–6.

Nugus, D. and Stokes, J.A. (2007). Bridging the gap: 15 years of service development and delivery: a model for community-based services in the UK. *Grief Matters: The Australian Journal of Grief and Bereavement*, **10**(2), 36–41.

O'Connell, B. (1998). *Solution-Focused Therapy*. London: Sage.

O'Hanlon, B. (2003). *A Guide to Inclusive Therapy: 26 Methods of Respectful Resistance-dissolving Therapy*. New York: Norton.

Rees, I. (2008). A systemic solution-oriented model. In B. Kelly, L. Woolfson, and J. Boyle (eds), *Frameworks for Practice in Educational Psychology: A Textbook for Trainees and Practitioners*. London: Jessica Kingsley, 162–82.

Renzenbrink, I. (2004). Relentless self-care. In J. Berzoff and P.R. Silverman (eds), *Living With Dying: A Handbook for End of Life Healthcare Practitioners*. New York: Columbia University Press.

Rogers, C. (1951). *Client-Centred Therapy: Its Current Practice, Implications and Theory*. London: Constable.

Rosenfeld, M., Seferiadis, A., Carlsson, J., and Gunnarsson, R. (2003). Active intervention in patients with whiplash-associated disorders improves long-term prognosis: A randomized controlled clinical trial. *Spine*, **28**(22), 2491–8.

Salloum, K. and Rynearson, E.K. (2006). Family resilience after violent death. In E.K. Rynearson (ed.), *Violent Death: Resilience and Intervention Beyond the Crisis*. New York: Routledge.

Schuurman, D. (2003). *Never the Same: Coming to Terms with the Death of a Parent*. New York: St. Martin's Press.

Selekman, M.D. (1997). *Solution-Focused Therapy with Children: Harnessing Family Strengths for Systemic Change*. New York: Guilford Press.

Silverman, P.R. (2000). *Never Too Young to Know: Death in Children's Lives*. New York: Oxford University Press.

Simon, J. (2010). *Solution Focused Practice in End-of-Life and Grief Counselling*. New York: Springer.

Stebnicki, M.A. (2007). Empathy fatigue: Healing the mind, body, and spirit of professional counsellors. *American Journal of Psychiatric Rehabilitation*, **10**(4), 317–38.

Stokes, J.A. (2004). *Then, Now and Always: Supporting Children as They Journey Through Grief*. Cheltenham: Winston's Wish.

Stroebe, M. and Schut, H. (1999). The dual process model for coping with bereavement: Rationale and description. *Death Studies*, **23**(3), 197–224.

Stubbs, D., Alilovic, K., Stokes, J.A., and Howells, K. (2006) *Family Assessment: Guidelines for Child Bereavement Practitioners*. Cheltenham: Winston's Wish.

Stubbs, D., Nugus, D. and Gardner, K. (2008). *Hope Beyond the Headlines: Supporting a Child Bereaved Through Murder or Manslaughter*. Cheltenham: Winston's Wish.

Stubbs, D. and Stokes, J. (2008). *Beyond the Rough Rock: Supporting a Child Who Has Been Bereaved Through Suicide*. Cheltenham: Winston's Wish.

Tonkin, L. (1996). Growing around grief: Another way of looking at grief and recovery. *Bereavement Care*, **15**(1), 10.

Vanistendael, S. (2008). We smile when life does not: Humour, resilience and spirituality: A summary reflection. Unpublished paper. Available at stefan.vanistendael@bice.org.

Vauth, R., Kleim, B., Wirtz, M., and Corrigan, P.W. (2007). Self-efficacy and empowerment as outcomes of self-stigmatizing and coping in schizophrenia. *Psychiatry Research*, **150**(1), 71–80.

Wheeler, J. (2008). A solution focused approach to bereavement. *Counselling Children and Young People, BACP*, June, 3.

Worden, J.W. (2009). *Grief Counseling and Grief Therapy: A Handbook for the Mental Health Practitioner*, 4th edn. New York: Springer.

Wortman, C.B. and Silver, R.C. (1989). The myths of coping with loss. *Journal of Consulting and Clinical Psychology*, **57**(3), 349–57.

Chapter 12

Compassion: the essence of end-of-life care

Philip Larkin

Introduction

> After the months in bed, Those Sundays to Fridays, Waiting for the morphine
> After the days and weeks of the kept-up face for her sisters and brother
> After the last words to her daughter and son, Nurse came to lay her out.
> At the loneliest moment, she sings a fragile lullaby, each note a petal of comfort.
> She was then mother of the world, rocking her baby to sleep, after the pain that
> was prayer
>
> ('Nurse', by Ned Crosby; reprinted with permission)

For those who work in palliative and end-of-life care, the words of Ned Crosby, a County Clare-based poet and Roman Catholic priest, resonates with the profound experience of being part of the dynamic between carer and cared-for at the moment of death. Understanding the dimensions of expert palliative care nursing reflects the need to balance the science and artistry of nursing to provide a framework in which dying becomes the culmination of a life well-lived and not a life transition to be feared (Ferrell and Coyle 2010; Larkin 2009). Nursing contributes one small part to the experience of care at end-of-life and yet, in acknowledging the role of others in this care setting, there is a unique element to the relationship of nursing to dying. Metaphors of journeying with, being present to, tending, holding, and nurturing all signify that aspect of what is needed clinically as people die comes from within (Seno, 2010; Sasser and Pulchalski, 2010; Mount et al., 2007; Boston and Mount, 2006; Henderson, 2001; Spall, 2001). The craft of end-of-life care implies that at some level an inner conscience governs our clinical discernment on what is fundamentally the right thing to do. In palliative care terms, this may be a decision to act or not act in a certain circumstances, a decision based on the wisdom of acknowledging our essential humility in face of the Natural Law of living and dying. This innate wisdom echoes a beautiful Talmudic phrase 'qol dmamah dagah—the voice of fragile silence', an inner voice which is an intangible yet consistent element of our being (Heschel, 1955). Understanding that this wisdom exists within us enables a reconfiguration of how we approach our clinical work with dying people. There has been an attempt to incorporate some of these deeper elements into the debate on caring versus curing, most visibly in medical literature and led by eminent physicians from palliative care, such as Balfour Mount, Michael Kearney, William Breitbart, and Eric Cassell (Kearney et al., 2009; Kearney, 2009; Cassell, 2009;

Breitbart, 2008; Mount and Kearney, 2003; Kearney, 2000). One such element which receives increasing attention is compassion.

Compassion 'provides the unspoken language to address unspeakable suffering' (Sasser and Puchalski, 2010, p. 937). Compassion is often described as an assumed quality within palliative care, and yet it remains under-researched and ill-defined in that context. Emphasis within current health literature would tend to focus on the idea of *compassion fatigue*, a syndrome describing the effect of being witness to the traumatic experience of other people and noted as a particular issue in palliative and end-of-life care (Showalter, 2010; Geller et al., 2010; Sabo, 2008; Wright, 2004; Figley, 1995). Although an important topic, what may be equally important is to describe and interpret as far as possible what true compassion means in the context of death and dying and how it underpins the approach to clinical engagement with dying people. Interpreting the influence of compassion in clinicians' thinking and motivations enables a new dialogue to take place around the complex practice of palliative and end-of-life care which often incorporates ethical, philosophical, and theological constructs.

As I write this chapter, the world is living through a time of unprecedented global economic crisis. Ireland, as a small agricultural country of 4.5 million people, has been at the forefront of this crisis. Having enjoyed significant years of prosperity (the 'Celtic Tiger' economy), it is now all too clear that this prosperity was based upon false economics. Today, rising unemployment, home repossession, and public and private sector salary cuts are indicators of the stress factors which impinge on the daily lives of Irish people. Emigration, which has determined the Irish experience since the mid-nineteenth century, has a profound effect on how Ireland both perceives itself and has been perceived by others (Dunne, 2003). Current data from the Central Statistics Office (2010) says the number of emigrants from Ireland in the year to April 2010 is estimated to have grown by over 40 per cent, from 45,300 to 65,100.

Palliative and end-of-life care has not been immune to these stressors. Cost reductions and reduced staffing levels impact on how staff perceive the delivery and quality of their caring and their personal self-worth as carer. Given the emotional intensity of the work and the factors noted here, there is every reason for people to experience the compassion fatigue described above. Yet there is something which sustains Irish palliative care practitioners to remain motivated and compassionate in their caring and which enables them to be present to the needs of dying people even in the current adverse situation.

In this chapter, I will argue that in order to understand issues such as compassion fatigue, it is really necessary to understand first what compassion is and in particular how compassion frames the essence of care at end-of-life. This will be discussed from the philosophical, ethical, and theological perspectives noted earlier, and situated in exemplars from research into the transition experiences of palliative care patients in the last weeks and months of life (Larkin et al., 2007a; Larkin et al., 2007b). A case will be made that the ability to articulate personal understanding of compassion enables palliative care practitioners to address the stressors of their clinical practice in a meaningful and productive way. First, it is necessary to clarify the context from which twenty-first-century palliative and end-of-life care is derived and the then the challenges faced by its practitioners today.

Palliative and end-of-life care: historical reflections on compassionate care

Case 1: Martin

Martin was a 78-year-old man with advanced cancer of the prostate. He had spent much of his adult life as a migrant labourer in England. He came back to Ireland to live with his sister from whom he had been estranged for many years and who died within two years of his coming home. He was admitted to the hospice for symptom management and it quickly became clear that he would stay in the hospice until he died. He responded to this decision positively: 'so many have died well here cared for by the Sisters. Now it is my turn, too.'

Although the contemporary history of palliative and hospice care is discussed elsewhere in this book, it is important to reflect back on its roots in the work of eighteenth- and nineteenth-century religious orders who instigated the vision of compassionate care for the sick and dying. To do this, I draw on two examples to show how compassion shaped the mission of two religious orders: the Irish Sisters of Charity in Ireland and the 'Grey Nuns' (Sisters of Charity of Montreal) in Canada. I choose these because both have subsequently influenced the founders of the hospice movement internationally. In her own letters, Cicely Saunders acknowledged how her early clinical experiences with the Irish Sisters of Charity in St Joseph's Hospice, Hackney, had a profound influence on her vision for the foundation of St Christopher's Hospice in Sydenham, London, ostensibly the first modern hospice (Saunders, 2005; Clark, 2002). The importance of her Christian faith in relation to her interpretation of palliative care will be discussed later. In Canada, palliative care physicians Eduardo Bruera and Balfour Mount both acknowledge the work of the Grey Nuns in establishing the services from which the transition from the hospice to palliative care movement developed. Their respective contribution to the development of health and social care provision in Ireland and Canada is well documented.

The response of Mother Mary Aikenhead, Foundress of the Irish Sisters of Charity to the Irish cholera epidemic of 1832 offers a good example of this (Fenning, 2003). It is estimated that over 50,000 died in Ireland from the cholera epidemic by the end of that year alone. Grangegorman prison in Dublin had been re-opened as a temporary hospital to house the sick and dying and the local authorities had approached the Sisters of Charity based in Stanhope Street and Gardiner Street for help. Conditions in the prison were extremely over-crowded with up to 80 patients dying per day. Since the risk of infection was high, the sisters would wash in chlorate of lime every night to keep any danger of infection away from the other nuns. As Fenning (2003) notes, the work of the Sisters in caring for the dying at that time was acknowledged in the local press:

> '1833, 15 Nov, The Sisters of Charity: During the frightful visitation of the cholera, the services rendered by these ladies to the cause of humanity surpass all praise (FJ 15 Nov)' (Fenning, 2003, p. 124).

The experience of the cholera epidemic persuaded Mother Aikenhead to set up St Vincent's Hospital, the first public hospital staffed and run by women in Ireland, in 1834.

The opening of Our Lady's Hospice, Harold's Cross, in 1879 fulfilled a long-held ambition of the Order to provide institutional care for the dying which continues today (O'Brien and Clark, 2005). As Martin's case highlights, for the people of Dublin, dying well is associated with the Irish (now Religious) Sisters of Charity. It is recorded that on the death of Mary Aikenhead, local workmen came to ask if they could have the honour to carry her coffin to the chapel.

The Canadian example from the same period has an interesting historical link to Ireland as evidenced in the response of the Montreal-based 'Grey Nuns' (founded in 1737 by Marguerite Dufrost de Lajemmerais d'Youville) to the plight of Irish famine refugees who arrived in Grosse Ile in Quebec in 1847–8 suffering from Typhus. The then Mother Superior, Mother McMullen, described the suffering of the sick and dying they nursed in the fever sheds: 'Those who thus cry aloud in their agony are strangers, but their hands are outstretched for relief . . . ' (http://www.qfhs.ca/lib_connart3.html).

The 6,000 who died are commemorated by a granite memorial at Pointe StCharles, the largest famine grave outside Ireland.

The religious foundation of healthcare is therefore of profound consideration in understanding the development of palliative care and in understanding why compassion is integral to its practice. Sevensky (1983) proposes nine core religious ideals which underpin the work of religions in healthcare. These include stewardship (the idea that we are put on earth to mind and care for), human dignity, the sanctity of life, justice, love or compassion, and finitude (that is, as humans, there are limitations to what we can do). These ideals echo ethical values which are ascribed to good medical practice and upon which the 'principalist' model of ethics in healthcare is built (Randall and Downie, 2006). However, Sevensky argues that the influence of these religious values are often subjugated to the narrative of medicine which is largely a secular activity based on experiment and empiricism. The religious care model went beyond cure-orientated medicine to the compassionate relief of illness and suffering. Of course, such values embrace all the living religions of the world, as well as having reference to the ancient Greco-Roman concepts of healing as in the temple of Aeskelpios, which has found a place in contemporary reflections on palliative care (Kearney, 2000). Overall, there is marked attention to the whole person, body, mind, and spirit, which challenges us to consider the basis of human existence. The idea that love is a motivating factor in the work of these early religious orders is one that does not always sit easily in modern descriptions of healthcare, but love clearly influenced the approach of religions in providing care for the sick and dying. One good example of this is offered by Connell Meehan (2003) in her description of 'careful nursing' as a model for contemporary practice. The concept of love has been further investigated in relation to nursing (Fitzgerald and van Hooft, 2000), sometimes expressed as charity (*Caritas*). Love and charity reflect both the motto of the Irish Sisters of Charity, '*Caritas Christi Urget Nos*' (the love of Christ urges us on) and the description of Marguerite d'Youville as ' Mother of Universal Charity' at her canonization by John XXIII in 1959. These examples are not unique and there are equally strong contemporaneous accounts of other religious orders caring for sick and dying people, especially in Ireland (Connell Meehan, 2003). They do, however, demonstrate an important factor in the description of compassion as a concept; that a compassionate response to suffering is through action and not merely an empathetic feeling towards others' misfortune.

Palliative and end-of-life care: contemporary reflections

Case 2: Pearl

Pearl was a 66-year-old West Indian woman with a spinal tumour. She was admitted to the hospice until a place of care could be arranged. Pearl described her admission to the hospice. 'I never knew. They never told me it was, you know, the hospice. They kept saying palliatative caring—I didn't know what they meant. They said they would take care of me, but I can't stay here now. I am going somewhere else.'

Naturally, it is important to consider how far these ideals of compassion and love, however defined, are visible in palliative and end-of-life care today. Pearl's story is not unique and would be familiar to many palliative care practitioners. The idea of palliative and end-of-life care as an institutionally based model of care until death is changing. Contemporary debate on end-of-life care questions whether 'palliative' care still embraces the original ideals of '*hospitium*' as a place of compassionate care and comfort at end-of-life or, if it has become a medically orientated discipline, focusing primarily on interventions for the relief of pain and other symptoms through any or all extraneous means. Death and dying is now seen as a part of the larger continuum of care with indistinct and blurred boundaries regarding the curative and active management of disease. Clearly, the World Health Organization (2002) revision of the definition of palliative care would favour this in its view of palliative and end-of-life care as applicable to a wide range of chronic and life-limiting illness. It is noted, however, that this redefinition is itself not without criticism (Randall and Downie, 2006). The shift in language to describe the various possibilities for the transition from living to dying (for example, curative, chronic, and life-limiting, supportive care, palliative care, end-of-life care, terminal care, etc.) suggests that when people now refer to palliative care, it is no longer clear what they mean with respect to death and dying (Illhardt, 2001). This does not preclude compassion occurring within a palliative care context but may make the unique work less visible in terms of how that care is delivered and how practitioners may support their patients and themselves to understand that 'through acceptance of the life one has lived comes acceptance of death' (Breitbart, 2008, p. 212).

This conceptual transition provides a significant point of stress for practitioners in terms of articulating their belief in what palliative care is and their motivation for staying in the field. Framing palliative care only in terms of its symptom management brief obscures the important role of the hospice as place of refuge which offers ontological security as death approaches (Heidegger, 1971/1992). The hospice space offers the opportunity for preparation and protection; time and energy devoted to the closing of life commitments, reflection on life relationships and ensuring the safety of family in practical and emotional terms. Unlike space as territory which is something bounded and closed, a hospice dwelling space represents something fluid and responsive, somewhere which nurtures a compassionate response and thus a positive outcome for people experiencing loss in their lives. (Larkin, 2007a; Gilmour, 2006; Williams, 2002; Young et al., 2002; MacGregor Wise, 2000). Hospices are a beacon to other centres of healthcare which are rapidly becoming impersonal, clinical out-patient-driven non-places (Milligan, 2003; Augé, 1995; Heidegger, 1971/1992; Bollnow, 1961). Perhaps the loss of soul in these buildings is a contributory factor to the experience of compassion fatigue.

Interpreting compassion: a prerequisite for caring at end of life

Case 3: Elizabeth

Elizabeth was a 48-year-old woman with a brain tumour. She had lived with her partner and his two children from a previous relationship for 11 years. One day, he told her that he could no longer care for her and his children and she would have to go. That evening, she arrived at the hospice unannounced with two suitcases, confused, disorientated, and with nowhere to go. She never saw her ex-partner or the children again.

Elizabeth's story is one which evokes many responses: shock, anger, disbelief, and of course compassion. Assuming that compassion is an important element in achieving a positive experience of life closure for patients and their relatives, a description of compassion as applied to a hospice/palliative care context is needed. Compassion has been described in terms of developing kindness towards all life and being able to face personal vulnerability in order to support others who are themselves vulnerable (Remen, 2000). The etymological definition of compassion arising from *com* (together with) and *pati* (to suffer) (*Oxford English Dictionary*, 2004) resonates with the ideals of palliative care in responding to suffering in a way that involves a partnership approach to working with something very visible but at the same time intangible. Schantz (2007) describes compassion as holding its own intrinsic moral and spiritual values. Compassion shares a critical element with palliative and end-of-life care: relationship. Compassion assumes that we have regard and respect for another human being, that we hold concern for the welfare of others, are aware of the nature of suffering, and have a desire to relieve that suffering if at all possible (Bergum, 2004; Bergum, 2003; Pask, 2003; Blum, 1980). For Cicely Saunders, relationship was demonstrated through close involvement in the unique personhood of the individual and their family as they lived through their experience of final illness (Randall and Downie, 2006). This prop-osition challenged the hierarchical model of doctor–patient relationship and to that extent was revolutionary in its thinking. Contemporary nursing scholars have suggest-ed that it is an imperative for nurses to engage in relationships with those they care for in order to meet the essence of clinical practice (Scott, 1998). There are many examples of the importance of relationship in palliative and end-of-life care literature, particu-larly from the perspective of the nurse (Ferrell, 2006; Abma, 2005; Brannström et al., 2005; Johns, 2004; Garnet, 2003). The shift in palliative medicine towards this more self-reflective and holistic model of practice is also acknowledged (Breitbart, 2008; Mount and Kearney, 2003).

Compassion may be seen in oneself as a positive moral emotion or evaluated positively by others who observe the quality. It is associated with other constructs such as fatigue, resilience, and love and is clearly perceived as a central tenet of nursing (Sabo, 2008; Alkema et al., 2008; Sabo, 2006; Randall and Downie, 2006; Pask, 2001; von Dietze and Orb, 2000). It has been described as the 'groundwork' of caring itself (Churchill, 1977).

Compassion raises an interesting challenge to the construct of empathy. Empathy has been widely adopted as the *sine qua non* for communication-skills training programmes in healthcare. It has recently been criticized for its use and misinterpretation in healthcare, notably because the objective stance it purports may distance the practitioner from the emotive nature of the other's situation, and, as we have noted, the willingness to engage with the other at this deep level is fundamental to compassion (Hayward, 2005; Jull, 2001). Empathy as a way of entering into the suffering of others can only be considered the beginning of what is needed for true compassion to exist (Dalai Lama, 2005). On the other hand, sympathy is usually considered an inappropriate professional response because of its connotations with pity and the loss of professional objectivity. Pity receives critical attention in the literature, particularly in the critique of philosopher Martha Nussbaum (Gallagher, 2009; Deigh, 2004; Nussbaum, 2001).

Linking pity and sympathy may well be erroneous in the context of compassion. Smith (1976) concludes that whereas we can be sympathetic to a range of emotions and situations, compassion and pity are only directed towards the sorrow of others. Both Christian and Buddhist perspectives would agree that compassion and pity are not synonymous. Barad (2007) argues that if pity and compassion were the same, everyone would experience both in equal measure, which is clearly not the case. Aquinas's treatise, *Summa Theologica*, makes a strong differentiation between compassion and pity that is resonant with contemporary clinical practice. He argues that pity as an emotional response can be harmful because it does not sufficiently acknowledge the importance of reason and choice in the demonstration of compassion. The compassionate person working from a place of reason is able to assist the sufferer in identifying solutions to problems. The Dalai Lama concurs with this, arguing that wisdom is essential to ensure that true compassion is ' put to the use of others' (Dalai Lama, 2006; Aquinas, 1981). Whether reason or wisdom equates with empathy needs further discussion. Suffice it to say, pity has a place in understanding compassion and how it is enacted.

Nussbaum (2001) defines three components to compassion. The first is a belief that the suffering undergone by the other person is significant. The second is that the suffering was, by and large, unmerited. Thirdly, for compassion to occur, the person who views the suffering must see that it has the potential to be experienced personally. There are, of course, caveats to all of these. For example, to what extent is the significance of suffering culturally derived? Is compassion different where the suffering is to some extent self-inflicted (for instance, the person with terminal lung cancer associated with a lifetime of cigarette smoking). Gallagher (2009) reflects on these questions in his discussion of tragedy, compassion, and forgiveness, a language noted in end-of-life care (the tragedy of loss, the need for forgiveness, etc.). He argues that even though the suffering may be hard to concretize, 'Compassion responds to the pain it can see with its eyes, and its natural expression is the embrace of care' (Gallagher, 2009, p. 239).

Nussbaum cites a fourth constituent to compassion, '*Eudaimonia*', sometimes translated as 'flourishing happiness'. The argument offered is that compassion occurs when well-being is considered in the context of mutuality. In other words, my well-being is affected by the suffering of others close to me. If it is assumed that palliative care nurses develop this close relationship along Cicely Saunders' ideals, then the concomitant risks of sadness and pain are evident. Of course, as in any philosophical discourse, there are opposing arguments. If *Eudaimonia* is based on relationship, how do we explain a compassionate response to suffering which is more remote? (Gallagher, 2009). Is the compassion we experience towards the victims of the recent earthquake in Haiti qualitatively different to that we experience at home with family and friends? Compassion is not innate since we make the choice to be compassionate or not (Schantz, 2007; Gyatso, 2002; Gyatso, 2001). Compassion also implies the idea of service to others and so is inadvertently associated with subservience or weakness. This may reflect the empathy/sympathy dichotomy noted earlier. It is possible to see in this brief discussion not only the complexity of compassion but how it may be linked to the care of dying people. Nussbaum's elements can be seen through the daily work of palliative care nurses in being present to the suffering of their patients (Abma, 2005; Johns, 2004). Yet the consequences of compassionate care and the impact of such on the caregiver are also well documented (Vachon and Müeller, 2009; Fillion et al., 2009; Asai et al, 2007; Vachon, 1995; Bram and Katz, 1989).

Compassion at end-of-life: a Christian reflection

You are the difference you make. (Nouwen et al., 1982)

It is interesting to note the trend towards Buddhist perspectives on compassion in both contemporary academic publications and 'self-help' literature that relates to the field of death, dying, and end-of-life care (Halifax, 2008; Fox, 1999). This is not surprising since compassion is the essence of Mahayana Buddhism (Dalai Lama, 1997). However, given that Cicely Saunders was a woman of strong Christian conviction (Clark, 2002), the modern basis of hospice and palliative care is essentially a Christian one. Cicely Saunders' early thoughts on how to develop care for the dying were shaped by her encounters with Olive Wyon, a theologian, her visits to the Sisters of the Communauté de Grandchamp, Switzerland, and of course her work with the Irish Sisters of Charity. She also envisaged the formation of a lay Christian community as the genesis of the movement (Clark, 2002). Therefore, from the perspective of palliative care, a different worldview may be required in order to interpret compassion in that particular context. This is not to say that hospice and palliative care was intended to be exclusively Christian. Cicely Saunders was equally clear that hospice was open to all, irrespective of religion. Rather, there may be elements within the Christian discussion on compassion, which add to the deeper understanding of what hospice and palliative care is.

Barad (2007) explores both Christian and Buddhist views of compassion from the viewpoint of Thomas Aquinas (1225–74) and His Holiness, the Fourteenth Dalai Lama. Aquinas's *Summa Theologica* addresses the elements of compassion through his discourse on charity (*caritas*) and mercy (*misericordia*). He argues that charity (*caritas*) is a theological virtue which leads to compassion. Mercy (*misericordia*) comes from the idea of the compassionate heart (*miserium cor*) responding to another's unhappiness. Although it is an interesting observation that whereas mercy is usually directed towards someone who has committed a wrong, compassion makes no such claim, Aquinas argues that in real terms compassion and mercy are synonymous. Interestingly, Buddhist teachings echo many of those of Aquinas relative to compassion and suffering, despite other theological differences. Aquinas argues that love is the most fundamental act of *caritas*. The importance of Caritas as a motivating factor in the compassionate acts of religions involved in the care of the dying has been noted already. Aquinas goes on to describe peace and joy as interior effects of *caritas*. This has an important message for practitioners since it states that compassion evokes peacefulness which can be sensed by others and lead to their increased sense of peace. In effect, 'compassion is contagious' (Barad, 2007, p. 21). Many of these ideals can be seen in the mission of the religious in working with the dying, as noted earlier in this chapter (Connell Meehan, 2003).

A more contemporary Christian reflection on compassion notes:

> Compassion asks us to go where it hurts, to enter into places of pain, to share in broken-ness, fear confusion and anguish . . . Compassion means full immersion in the condition of being human. (Nouwen et al., 1982, p. 4)

Nouwen et al. (1982) argue that depth of feeling evoked by compassion is evidenced in its Greek translation, '*splangchnizomai*', something felt deep within the gut. Compassion is not simply about achieving a satisfactory outcome. Compassion requires action and has limited value if it does not lead to activity designed to respond to another's suffering. Compassion also has a strong community-orientated message for social justice, particularly in relation to the compassionate presence of someone supporting another's struggle (Vachon and Huggard, 2010; Nussbaum, 2001; Nouwen et al., 1982). This depth of feeling would resonate with Cicely Saunders' own belief that 'the way care is given can reach the most hidden places' (Saunders, 1996). In this, she argues that our humanity and vulnerability hold equal importance to our professional competence. Compassion is about believing in one's personal capacity and innate qualities to address the pain and suffering of this world, beyond religious language and practice which reflects the view that 'You are the difference you make' (Nouwen et al., 1982).

Compassion in action: a relational-ethical dialogue for palliative care practice

Case 4 Kathleen

Kathleen was a 48-year-old woman with advanced ovarian cancer admitted to the hospice for end-of-life care. Her husband Tony was already an in-patient in the hospice. Tony died two days after Kathleen was admitted. The impact of caring for both Kathleen and Tony was evident from clinical case review meetings. Staff expressed their pain and sadness over the unique situation of caring for a husband and wife at the same time. They struggled with the sense of injustice that their young children should lose both parents so close together. They felt a need to create an environment of care which could absorb the distress of the family and of each other. This was 'one of those cases.'

In this final section, I will try to draw some of the theoretical components discussed into a reflection on how an understanding of compassion in action can transform the way in which we care for people at end-of-life. Kathleen's case needs to be set against a background of the economic downturn in Ireland. At the time of Kathleen's admission, all public sector workers, including the hospice nursing staff, had taken a significant cut in salary, leading to a general sense of frustration and demoralization with professional life. Caring for Kathleen, both as a dying patient and a recent widow, gave rise to a deeper reflection within the team on the purpose and focus of that life. Some of this focused back on issues cited earlier; the shifting dynamic of palliative care, the motivation to stay in a complex and emotionally challenging field, and also the complexity of providing compassionate care in a system that is predominantly business-orientated, consumerist, and with an emphasis on measurement and outcome. The need to re-focus is evident from initiatives such as the Compassion in Healthcare movement (www.compassioninhealthcare.org), which advocates for just, moral, and ethical approaches to patient care (Youngson, 2008; Chew et al., 2003). Addressing this warrants a two-fold approach. Self-care is certainly one way in which the stress of compassionate caring can be assuaged (Kearney et al., 2009). There is some evidence that palliative care practitioners derive strength from their work at the existential level and, indeed, through the very patient–professional relationship which can of itself drain personal resources (Kearney, 2009; Boston and Mount, 2006). A second approach is based on the fundamental premise of this chapter: compassion as relationship. To do this, I return to Ned Crosby's poem at the beginning of this chapter and look to the writing of another Irish poet and philosopher, John O'Donohue (1956–2008) to frame a discussion on compassionate nursing as an interpretation of relational ethics.

The possibilities offered by a relational ethics approach to care for nursing have been explored and with reference to palliative care and suffering (Abma, 2005; Fredriksson and Eriksson, 2003; Fredriksson and Eriksson, 2001; Fredriksson, 1999; Gadow, 1999). The Canadian scholars Vangie Bergum and John Dossetor (2000) speak of relational ethics as a way to enhance 'human flourishing (*eudaimonia*) through healthy and ethical relationships', a concept already shown to have reference to compassion (Nussbaum, 2001). Relational ethics challenges the 'four-principle' approach of bio-medical ethics which always seeks universal and impartial judgements to be made. It focuses on the commitment that exists between persons, the emotive nature of relationship, and the context of environment in determining just actions. To this end, relational ethics offers a practice-based and action-orientated approach to complex decision-making (Bergum and Dossetor, 2000). Relational ethics would give substance to the concept of intuition. There is little written on intuition in palliative care nursing research, although it would have a strong place in the language of nurses in practice. This may be due to the dichotomy between the science and art of nursing, with the former dominant model in healthcare negating the practice wisdom derived from the latter (Larkin, 2009). Yet, for nurses like those in Crosby's poem, what they do at this vital transition is derived from something more than diagnostic reasoning, and in this brief reflection on Bergum and Dossetor's (2000) relational ethics framework, I interpret compassion as the motivation for this nurse as 'mother of the world, rocking her baby to sleep.'

The ideal of *embodiment* considers that connection, however brief, can be meaningful at the deepest level. The encounter between these two women, one carer, the other cared-for, is not based on time, but rather presence. In that moment, led by the compassion which frames the nurse's reason for being present to this dying woman in the first place, she (the nurse) seems to understand what is fundamentally expected of her at this time–to guide the patient and family safely from living to dying. O'Donohue (2003) describes the deathbed as a 'a place of intense energy' (p. 203). The ability to attend and be present to dying would shape the compassionate response offered by the nurse to her patient and the family.

Engagement arises when we enable the emotional aspects of a person's life to take precedence over our (the clinician's) need for objectivity as the judge of good care. There is a great affinity between Crosby's metaphorical description of the nurse's work at the moment of death as a 'fragile lullaby' and the image of '*qol dmamah dagah*–the voice of fragile silence', noted earlier (Heschel, 1955). Both speak of the hidden language compassion evokes in terms of knowing what is intuitively the right thing to do or say.

Mutual respect demands an acknowledgement of uniqueness and individuality. The procedure of 'laying-out' is the final act of compassionate care that can be given by the nurse to their patient. Through their connection, the nurse may have learnt of the 'broken, empty spaces' (O'Donohue, 2003, p. 194) which have been a part of their patients' life and in some way may have touched those of her own life. The tenderness exhibited in the nurse laying-out her patients bears witness to the humanity and vulnerability which encapsulates true compassion.

Bergum and Dossetor (2000, p. xiii) conclude that *environment* exists in a ' web of relations' and that we need to understand how the individual exists within this to be able to see the real person. O'Donohue (2003), in common with other philosophers, acknowledges that the home is not a building but a shelter of intimacy and love. In entering the home, the nurse creates a 'relational space' which protects the intimacy of loss and grief and enables a sharing of memory about the dead woman. Her actions highlight how 'the beauty of compassion continues to shelter and save our world' (O'Donohue, 2003, p. 181).

Conclusion

This chapter has only offered a brief reflection on the possibilities that compassion brings to the understanding of end-of-life care. There are, indeed, many other philosophical and theological interpretations of compassion that could be used to deepen the discussion. Interpreting the consequences of compassionate caring requires firstly an understanding of compassion itself. There is, for example, a contemplative element to compassion which is resonant with death and dying: the ability to embrace stillness and silence. This warrants further discussion. Ireland has a long and distinguished history in caring compassionately for dying people and that history has shaped what we currently consider dying well. In a final reflection, John O'Donohue contends that 'no-one was sent into the world without being given the infinite possibilities of the heart' (O'Donohue, 2003, p. 244). Compassion arises from the ability to use that heart wisely in caring for others and knowing how and when to care for oneself. Compassion offers challenges and consolations but ultimately it asks us to consider what caring truly means.

References

Abma, T.A. (2005). Struggling with the fragility of life: A relational-narrative approach to ethics in palliative nursing. *Nursing Ethics*, **12**(4): 337–48.

Alkema, K., Linton, J., and Davies, R. (2008). A study of the relationship between self-care, compassion satisfaction, compassion fatigue, and burnout among hospice workers. *Journal of Social Work in End-of-Life and Palliative Care*, **4**, 101–19.

Aquinas T. (1981). *Summa Theologica*, trans. Fathers of the English Dominican Province. Westminster: Christian Classics.

Asai, M., Morita, T., Akechi, T, et al. (2007). Burnout and psychiatric morbidity among physicians engaged in end-of-life care for cancer patients: A cross-sectional nationwide survey in Japan. *Psycho-Oncology*, **16**, 421–8.

Augé, M. (1995). *Non-Places: An Introduction to an Anthropology of Supermodernity*, trans. John Howe. London: Verso.

Barad, J. (2007). The understanding and experience of compassion: Aquinas and the Dalai Lama. *Buddhist-Christian Studies*, **27**, 11–29.

Bergum, V. (2004). Relational ethics in nursing. In J. Storch, P. Rodney, and R. Starzomski (eds), *Toward a Moral Horizon: Nursing Ethics for Leadership and Practice*. Toronto: Prentice-Hall, 485–503.

Bergum, V. (2003). Relational pedagogy: Embodiment, improvisation and interdependence. *Nursing Philosophy*, **4**, 121–8.

Bergum, V. and Dossetor, J. (2000). *Relational Ethics: The Full Meaning of Respect*. Hagerstown, MD: University Publishing Group.

Blum, L. (1980). Compassion. In A.M. Rorty (ed.), *Explaining Emotions*. Berkeley, CA: University of California Press, 507–17.

Bollnow, O.F. (1961). Lived space. *Philosophy Today*, **5**, 31–9.

Boston, P.H, and Mount B.M. (2006). The caregiver's perspective on existential and spiritual distress in palliative care. *Journal of Pain and Symptom Management*, **32**(1), 13–26.

Bram, P.J. and Katz, L.F. (1989). Study of burnout in nurses working in hospice and hospital oncology settings. *Oncology Nursing Forum*, **16**, 555–60.

Brannström, M., Brulin, C., Norberg, A., Boman, K., and Strandberg, G. (2005). Being a palliative nurse for persons with severe congestive heart failure in advanced homecare. *European Journal of Cardiovascular Nursing*, **4**(4), 314–23.

Breitbart, W. (2008). Thoughts on the goals of psychosocial palliative care. *Palliative and Supportive Care*, **6**, 211–12.

Cassell, E.J. (2009). Suffering. In D. Walsh, A. Caraceni, K.M. Foley, P. Glare, et al. (eds), *Palliative Medicine*. Philadelphia: Saunders Elsevier, 46–51.

Chew, M., Armstrong, R.M., and Van der Weyden, M.B. (2003). Can compassion survive the 21st century? *Editorial Medical Journal of Australia*, **179**, 569–70.

Churchill, L. (1977). Ethical issues of a profession in transition. *American Journal of Nursing*, **77**(5), 873–5.

Clark, D. (ed.) (2002). *Cicely Saunders—Founder of the Hospice Movement, Selected Letters 1959–1999*. Oxford: Oxford University Press.

Connell Meehan, T. (2003). Careful nursing: A model for contemporary nursing practice. *Journal of Advanced Nursing*, **44**(1), 99–107.

Dalai Lama (1997). *The Heart of Compassion*. Twin Lakes, WI: Iona Press.

Dalai Lama (2005). *How to Expand Love: Widening the Circle of Loving Relationships*. New York: Atria Books.

Dalai Lama (2006). *Kindness, Clarity, Insight*. Ithaca, NY: Snow Lion publications.

Deigh, J. (2004). Nussbaum's account of compassion. *Philosophy and Phenomenological Research*, **68**(2), 465–72.

von Dietze, E. and Orb, A. (2000). Compassionate care: A moral dimension of nursing. *Nursing Inquiry*, **7**(3), 166–74.

Dunne, C. (2003). *An Unconsidered People: The Irish in London*. London: New Island.

Fenning, H. (2003). The cholera epidemic in Ireland 1832–3: Priests, ministers and doctors. *Archivium Hibernicum*, **57**, 77–125.

Ferrell, B.R. (2006). Understanding the moral distress of nurses witnessing medically futile care. *Oncology Nursing Forum*, **33**(5), 992–30.

Ferrell, B.R. and Coyle, N. (2010). *Oxford Textbook of Palliative Nursing*, 3rd edn. New York: Oxford University Press.

Figley, C.R. (ed.) (1995). *Compassion Fatigue: Coping with Secondary Traumatic Stress Disorder in Those Who Treat the Traumatized*. New York: Brunner/Mazel.

Fillion, L., Duval, S., Dumont, S., et al. (2009). Impact of a meaning-centered intervention on job satisfaction and on quality of life among palliative care nurses. *Psycho oncology*, **18**, 1300–10.

Fitzgerald, L. and van Hooft, S. (2000). A Socratic dialogue on the question 'What is love in nursing'? Nursing *Ethics*, **7**, 481–91.

Fox, M. (1999). *Spirituality Named Compassion: Uniting Mystical Awareness with Social Justice*. Rochester, VT: Inner Traditions.

Fredriksson, L. (1999). Modes of relating in a caring conversation: A research synthesis on presence, touch and listening. *Journal of Advanced Nursing*, **30**, 1167–76.

Fredriksson, L. and Eriksson, K. (2001). The patient's narrative of suffering—a path to health? An interpretive research synthesis on narrative understanding. *Scandinavian Journal of Caring Science*, **15**, 3–11.

Fredriksson, L. and Eriksson K. (2003). The ethics of the caring conversation. *Nursing Ethics*, **10**, 138–47.

Gadow, S. (1999). Relational narratives: The postmodern turn in nursing ethics. *Scholarly Inquiry in Nursing Practice*, **13**, 57–70.

Gallagher, P. (2009). The grounding of forgiveness: Martha Nussbaum on compassion and mercy. *American Journal of Economics and Sociology*, **68**(1), 231–52.

Garnet, M. (2003). Sustaining the cocoon: The emotional inoculation produced by complementary therapies in palliative care. *European Journal of Cancer Care*, **12**, 129–36.

Geller R., Krasner, M., and Korones, D. (2010). Clinician self-care: The application of mindfulness-based approaches in preventing professional burnout and compassion fatigue. *Journal of Pain and Symptom Management*, **39**(2), 366.

Gilmour, J.A. (2006). Hybrid space: Constituting the hospital as a home space for patients. *Nursing Inquiry*, **13**, 16–22.

Gyatso, G.K. (2002). *Universal Compassion: Inspiring Solutions for Difficult Times*. New York: Tharpa Publications.

Gyatso, T. (2001). The compassionate life, by the Dalai Lama. Retrieved 20 June 2010 from www.Shambhalasun.com/revolving_themes/HHDL/compassion.

Halifax, J. (2008). Being with dying: Cultivating compassion and fearlessness in the presence of death. New York: Shambala Publications.

Hayward, R. (2005). Empathy. *Lancet*, **366**, 1071.

Heidegger, M. (1971). Building dwelling thinking. In *Martin Heidegger, Basic Writings*, ed. D.F. Krell. San Francisco: Harper, 347–63.

Henderson, M.L. (2001). Living fully while dying. *Journal of Pain and Symptom Management*, **21**(4), 357–8.

Heschel, A.J. (1955). *God in Search of Man*. New York: Harper Torchbooks.

Illhardt, F.J. (2001). Scope and demarcation of palliative care. In H. Ten Have and R. Janssens (eds), *Palliative Care in Europe: Concepts and Policies*. Amsterdam: IOS Press, 109–16.

Johns, C. (2004). *Being Mindful, Easing Suffering: Reflections on Palliative Care*. London: Jessica Kingsley.

Jull, A. (2001). Compassion: A concept exploration. *Nursing Praxis in New Zealand Inc*, **1**, 16–23.

Kearney, M. (2000). *A Place of Healing: Working with Suffering in Living and Dying*. Oxford: Oxford University Press.

Kearney, M.K., Weininger, R.B., Vachon, M.L.S., Mount, B.M., and Harrison, R.L. (2009). Self-care of physicians caring for patients at the end of life: 'Being connected . . . a key to my survival'. *Journal of the American Medical Association*, **301**, 1155–64.

Kearney, M. (2009). *A Place of Healing: Working with Nature and Soul at the End of Life*. New Orleans: Spring Journal Books.

Larkin, P.J. (2009). Nurses and nurse practitioners. In D. Walsh, A. Caraceni, K.M. Foley, P. Glare et al. (eds), Palliative Medicine. Philadelphia: Saunders Elsevier, 265–69.

Larkin, P., Direckx de Casterlé, B., and Schotsmans, P. (2007a). Towards a conceptual analysis of transience in relation to palliative care. *Journal of Advanced Nursing*, **59**, 86–96.

Larkin, P., Direckx de Casterlé, B., and Schotsmans, P. (2007b). Transition towards end-of-life care: An exploration of its meaning for palliative care patients in Europe. *Journal of Palliative Care*, **23**(2), 69–79.

Macgregor Wise, J. (2000). Home: Territory and identity. *Cultural Studies*, **14**, 295–310.

Milligan, C. (2003). Location or dis-location? Toward a conceptualization of people and place in the care-giving experience. *Social and Cultural Geography*, **4**, 455–70.

Mount, B.M., Boston, P.H., and Cohen, S.R. (2007). Healing connections: On moving from suffering to a sense of well-being. *Journal of Pain and Symptom Management*, **33**(4), 372–88.

Mount, B. and Kearney, M. (2003). Healing and palliative care: Charting our way forward. *Palliative Medicine*, **17**, 657–8.

Nouwen, H.J.M., McNeill, D., and Morrison, D. (1982). *Compassion—A Reflection on the Christian life*. New York: Doubleday.

Nussbaum, M.C. (1994). *The Therapy of Desire: Theory and Practice in Hellenistic Ethics*. Princeton: Princeton University Press.

Nussbaum, M.C. (2001). *Upheavals in Thought: The Intelligence of Emotions*. Cambridge: Cambridge University Press.

O'Brien, T. and Clark, D. (2005). A national plan for palliative care: The Irish experience. In J. Ling and L. O'Siorain (eds), *Palliative Care in Ireland*. Facing Death Series. Berkshire: Open University Press, 3–18.

O'Donohue, J. (2003). *Divine Beauty: The Invisible Embrace*. London: Bantam Press.

Pask, E.J. (2001). Nursing responsibility and conditions of practice: Are we justified in holding nurses responsible for their behavior in situations of patient care? *Nursing Philosophy*, **2**, 42–52.

Pask, EJ. (2003). Moral agency in nursing: Seeing value in the work and believing that I make a difference. *Nursing Ethics*, **10**, 165–74.

Randall, F. and Downie, R.S. (2006). *The Philosophy of Palliative Care: Critique and Reconstruction*. Oxford: Oxford University Press.

Remen, R.N. (2000). *My Grandfather's Blessings*. New York: Riverhead Books.

Sabo, B. (2008). Adverse psychological consequences: Compassion fatigue, burnout and vicarious traumatization: Are nurses who provide palliative and haematological cancer care vulnerable? *Indian Journal of Palliative Care*, **14**, 23–9.

Sabo, B.M. (2006). Compassion fatigue in nursing work: Can we accurately capture the consequences of caring work? *International Journal of Nursing Practice*, **12**, 136–42.

Sasser, C.G. and Pulchalski, C.M. (2010). The humanistic clinician: Traversing the science and art of health care. *Journal of Pain and Symptom Management*, **39**(5), 936–40.

Saunders, C. (2005). Foreword. in J. Ling and L. O'Siorain (eds), *Palliative Care in Ireland*. Facing Death Series. Berkshire: Open University Press, xix–xxii.

Saunders C. (1996). Into the valley of the shadow of death: A personal therapeutic journey. *British Medical Journal*, **7072**(313), 1599–1601.

Schantz, M. (2007). Compassion: A concept analysis. *Nursing Forum*, **42**(2), 48–55.

Scott, A. (1998). Nursing, narrative and the moral imagination. In T. Greenhalgh and B. Hurwitz (eds), *Narrative-based Medicine*. London: BMJ Books.

Seno, V.L. (2010). Being with dying: Authenticity in end of life encounters. *American Journal of Hospice and Palliative Care OnlineFirst*, published 3 May 2010 as DOI: 10.1177/1049909109359628.

Sevensky, R.L. (1983). The religious foundations of health care: a conceptual approach. *Journal of Medical Ethics*, **9**, 165–9.

Showalter, S.E. (2010). Compassion fatigue: What is it? Why does it matter? Recognizing the symptoms, acknowledging the impact, developing the tools to prevent compassion fatigue and strengthen the professional already suffering from the effects. *American Journal of Hospice and Palliative Medicine*, **27**(4), 239–42.

Smith, A (1976). Foreword in Raphael D.D. and Macfie A.L. (1976) *A Theory of Moral Sentiments*. Oxford: Clarendon Press.

Spall, B., Read, S., and Chantry, D. (2001). Metaphor: Exploring its origins and therapeutic use in death, dying and bereavement. *International Journal of Palliative Nursing*, **7**(7), 345–53.

Vachon, M.L.S. (1995). Staff stress in palliative/hospice care: A review. *Palliative Medicine*, **9**, 91–122.

Vachon, M.L.S. and Huggard, J. (2010). The experience of the nurse in end-of-life care in the 21st century: Mentoring the next generation. In B.R. Ferrell and N. Coyle (eds), *The Oxford Textbook of Palliative Nursing*, 3rd edn. New York: Oxford University Press, 1131–55.

Vachon, M.L.S. and Mueller, M. (2009). Burnout and symptoms of stress. In W. Breitbart and H. Chochinov (eds), *Handbook of Psychiatry in Palliative Medicine*. New York: Oxford University Press, 559–625.

Williams, A. (2002). Changing geographies of care: Employing the concept of therapeutic landscape as a framework in examining home space. *Social Science & Medicine*, 55, 141–54.

World Health Organization (2002). Definition of palliative care. Retrieved 16 June 2010 from http://www.who.int/cancer/palliative/definition/en/print.html

Wright, B. (2004). Compassion fatigue: How to avoid it. *Palliative Medicine*, 18, 3–4.

Young, B., Dixon-Woods, M., Findlay, M., and Heney, D. (2002). Parenting in a crisis: Conceptualizing mothers of children with cancer. *Social Science and Medicine*, **55**, 1835–47.

Youngson, R. (2008). Compassion in healthcare: The missing dimension of healthcare reform. Futures Debate, the NHS Confederation, Paper 2. Downloaded 16 May 2010 from www.debatepapers.org.uk.

Chapter 13

Clinical supervision and reflective practice in palliative care: luxury or necessity?

Pam Firth

Introduction

One of the areas in palliative care lacking both research and practice development is clinical supervision. Clinical supervision is often highlighted as a necessity for good safe practice but is seen in most organizations as a luxury and by some practitioners as a threat. Despite directives particularly from UK nursing bodies, many organizations still do not have robust systems in place. Moreover where clinical supervision is available it can be a web of *ad hoc* internal and external arrangements which lack coherence and focus.

The chapter will examine some of the issues, refer to research, and describe some examples of organizational attempts to set up a service-wide model of supervision, including that developed by the author. The starting point will be to examine some definitions and the difference in professional approaches. The main approach of this chapter is to focus on clinical supervision being offered in a small group setting.

Definitions

Palliative care has traditionally been offered by multi-professional teams all of whom have different ethics, codes of practices, skills, and competencies, but all have the central need to communicate with patients and their families at a time of extreme stress and strain within the family system (Firth, 2006). Some palliative care professionals, mostly non-medical/nursing, have to have external supervision by accredited supervisors in order to meet the requirements for their professional accreditation, for example counsellors, psychotherapists, art therapists, psychologists, family therapists, and others. Some non-medical professionals may complain that the prefix *clinical* medicalizes the activity, but this is the common title used.

The issues of clinical supervision are also central to achieving clinical governance with the focus of making sure that in service provision there is a commitment to high-quality patient-centred care and safe practices (Bishop, 2007). Bishop and Sweeney (2006), quoted in Bishop(2007), offer the following definition which reflects the emphasis on quality.

> Clinical supervision is a designated interaction between two or more practitioners within a safe and supportive environment that enables a continuum of reflective critical analysis of care, to ensure quality patients services, and the well being of the practioner.

Bond and Holland (2001) point out that any definition will be incomplete, but they suggest that clinical supervision has to be regular, in protected time, and facilitated by an experienced practitioner who has expertise in supervision. Their emphasis again is on the achievement of high quality of practice and the development of the supervisee. They go further in suggesting that it is the agenda of the supervisee that leads the sessions, which in turn promotes the active commitment of the supervisees. The supervisee is expected to reflect on the part they play in the complexity of events.

Faugier (1996) supports the growth model, which is about empowerment not control and can be useful in reframing staff ideas. A great value of supervision is that it should be well facilitated and can provide a safe learning environment.

The creativity of the facilitator is an important factor in supporting growth in the practitioner not just clinically but also personally. There is a natural tension between individual and group needs. The similarity to an educator is the capacity to look at the training, competency, skills, and needs of the person, organization, and profession and to celebrate the development of the individual for the good of the patient and family.

The partnership concept is promoted by Proctor (1988) with her definition:

> Supervision is a working alliance between worker or workers, in which the workers can reflect on themselves in their working situation by giving an account of their work, and receiving feedback and, where appropriate, guidance.

The working alliance model familiar to counsellors is central to the idea of trust boundaries and attendance to the work. It also implies that supervision is a process.

Proctor's description of an integrated model (1988) is a valuable way to consider the stages and process of supervision borrowing concepts from the group work theory of Tuckman (1965), and is quoted below.

- *Formative* developing skills/understanding through reflection.
- *Normative* importance of professional and organizational standards.
- *Restorative* the supportive elements of supervision.

Developing the models including reflective practice

In any project the support of the management, and in the case of voluntary organizations the trustees as well, is a key to a good outcome. Every step has to be well thought through. The need for all clinical staff to agree to the aims and the development of a culture takes time and some financial backing. The following account is a description of the author's experience of leading and developing a system of clinical supervision for the multi-professional staff group in a medium-sized hospice serving an area that consisted of 5 small towns and 240 villages in the south-east of England.

The first task was to find out who had supervision and where from. The next step was to try to establish what people thought supervision was. The following quote from

Hawkins and Shoet (2000) was used to stimulate discussion about supervision and formed part of the questionnaire sent to all staff.

> In choosing to help, where our role is to pay attention to someone else's needs, we are entering into a relationship which is different from the normal and everyday. There are times when it barely seems worth-while, perhaps because we are battling against the odds, or because the client is ungrateful, or because we feel drained and seemingly have nothing left to give. In times of stress it is sometimes easy to keep one's head down, to 'get on with it' and not take time to reflect. Organisations, teams and individuals can collude with this attitude for a variety of reasons, including pressures and internal fears of exposing one's own inadequacies.

Feedback about the quote, which was included in the questionnaire, was scarce, so the assumption was of agreement. However, one person objected to the thought that they may not have anything else to give. However, all staff were keen to have clinical supervision and in multi-professional groups where possible.

The subsequent work was to organize training for staff and supervisors. The only feasible model would be to adopt small group approach because of the of the size of the clinical staff group.

Any small group situation engenders a range of issues such as the individual versus the group, as well as worries about trust and fair amount of competition. Groups challenge us in a way that individuals do not (Firth, 2005). In palliative care, group supervision can give participants permission to express a range of feelings if the facilitator is trained and understands the need for containment. We therefore arranged for a module on group work to be included in the training for supervisors.

Reflection and reflective practice are central to examining one's own practice. For some authors it takes the form of a reflective diary and for others (for example Johns (1994)) it is a much more structured way of reflection.

Freshwater (2007) uses ideas from Kolb (1984) about the circular way of learning through reflection which requires us to start from the awareness of uncomfortable feelings which have to be evaluated and critically analysed in order to achieve a new perspective. Is reflective practice at the heart of clinical supervision or are they two sides of the same coin (Freshwater, 2007)? The author believes that the two have been developed separately but belong together.

Different professional attitudes to clinical supervision

Social work has always been committed to supervision but it differs from most of the models offered in this chapter. Supervision has long been held as a cornerstone of the profession and therefore it carries no stigma for social workers (Reith and Payne, 2009), whereas many writers reflect that nurses are threatened by supervision (Bond and Holland, 2001). Social work supervision is the major way in which social workers are taught, given support, and managed. The manager is responsible for the supervision of the staff and thus case management often is the focus. Currently the huge pressure on statutory social work will ensure that this model will continue. This raises questions about power inequalities and the fact that many managers are not trained. Kadushin (1992) described social work supervision as being *educative*, *supportive*, and *managerial*.

However, most specialist palliative care social workers work in multi-professional teams where a nursing/medical model is dominant, and many in palliative care social work are dual trained and therefore choose to adopt the model of counselling supervision. The counselling models emphasize the importance of the boundaries of the sessions, such as confidentiality. Time and place are seen as important and consistent structures which help to contain feelings of the participants.

The need to separate out the management role from that of clinical supervisor is important if the supervision is to allow time for participants to reflect on strong feelings and for participants to feel safe to explore what might be seen as weaknesses. Many palliative care social workers have external supervision as well as that supplied by their manager.

Nursing has been slow to embrace clinical supervision although the the UK National Nursing and Midwifery Council (NMC) recommended clinical supervision in 2002 and suggested from its research that it had the following benefits:

◆ Safer practice.

◆ Reduction of untoward incidents and complaints.

◆ Better focusing of education and professional development.

◆ Better assessments.

◆ Reduced staff stress.

◆ Improved confidence and professional development.

◆ Improved levels of sickness and absenteeism.

◆ Greater awareness of accountability.

◆ Better input into management appraisal systems.

◆ Better managed risk and better awareness of evidence-based practice.

In 2005 the Nursing and Midwifery Council again stated that all nurses should have access to clinical supervision. Their definition is as follows:

> A practice focused professional relationship that enables you to reflect on your practice with the support of a skilled supervisor. Through reflection you can further develop your skills, knowledge and enhance your understanding of your own practice. (NMC, 2005)

The author in planning clinical supervision for the organization trained all staff in the central tenets of supervision. The work of Faugier (1996) was particularly helpful because the hospice management wanted to encourage an empowerment model. Training for supervisors was commissioned from a university palliative care nursing department and all potential supervisors received the same two-day training. Although many supervisors were already trained it was important that all supervisors work from the same model.

Doctors

Traditionally doctors have not sought supervision, although a series of supervision groups for GPs and community physicians organized in the 1970s by Balint at the Tavistock Clinic, UK, became famous for the development of a group of very psychologically aware doctors. The author currently holds weekly clinical supervision sessions for junior doctors. They are given encouragement and protected time to attend. The focus of the session is to give space for the doctors, new to palliative care and on placement for maximum of four months, to bring whatever they wish. Usually feelings about loss and bereavement are explored as well as ethical practice. The doctors are also introduced to research-based learning about the psychosocial issues of patients and their families.

Research

There is a paucity of research into the efficacy of clinical supervision. It is something that often falls off the research and conference agenda, and yet in services being set up following the NICE guidelines (2004) UK, called the *Guidance on Cancer Services: Improving Supportive Care for Adults with Cancer*, practitioners are encouraged to set up systems of supervision to support the competency levels of workers particularly in the field of psychology and bereavement care. (NICE stands for National Institute for Health and Clinical Excellence which provides guidance, sets quality standards, and manages a national database to improve people's health and prevent and treat ill health.)

Most of the applicable research can be found in the field of mental health nursing. Kelly et al. (2001) studied the clinical supervision of mental health nurses working in Northern Ireland. The main findings were the uncertainty about its value. There was an acknowledged muddle about models: whether it was about management, quality control versus the personal/professional interface.

The training of supervisors was found to be deficient and the meaning and purpose was unclear. However these results from the research were used in the Clinical Supervision for Mental Health Nurses in Northern Ireland—Best Practice Guide, published in 2005, where there was an acknowledgement of patchy development in Northern Ireland.

Edwards et al. (2005) studied the supervision of mental health nurses and found that longer sessions were rated higher and that supervision worked well where the supervisee could choose their supervisor. This would not be unusual in counselling supervision. Staff who were themselves trained in supervision valued supervision the most. A fascinating study by Hyrkas (2005) examined the supervision of all types of nursing in Finland and found that group supervision was less effective than individual supervision and that female staff rated supervision more highly than male staff (they took into account that nursing is in general a female-dominated profession). Older staff rated it more highly than younger staff and frequency was important.

Fletcher (2008), working in Australia, developed and evaluated a clinical supervision programme for community nurses that included palliative care nurses. Her model was derived from social work/counselling where the focus was on the counselling relationship. The supervisors were not nurses but social workers. Her findings suggest that there was potential to encourage interprofessional and multi-professional working. She observed that there was value in nurses learning to have counselling-type conversations with patients.

McCloskey and Taggart (2010)explored the occupational stress in children's hospice nurses. They discussed the dominant discourse in relationships and described the long, intense relationships staff had with the families of the children they cared for. They observed that the nurses were in touch with the draining of family coping skills and the effects on parents mental health. Attachment issues, anger, and blame were all recognized as being commonplace in the work. Exposure to poignant moments was also a feature of the work. They conclude that clinical supervision and debriefing are part of the requirements to care for nurses in this setting.

Two further models of implementing a clinical supervision programme for staff in a hospice setting

(A) Chilvers (2009) describes a process of implementing a clinical supervision programme for nurses across three hospices. In many ways it is similar to the system used by the author. In their situation the supervision was for trained nurses and healthcare assistants. They used a two-day course to train supervisors commissioned from a university and also trained all staff in a supervision awareness. They adopted a groupwork model and allocated six staff to each group. Emphasis on the choice of supervisor was based on personal qualities and skills. They produced a supervision policy. Also supervisees could choose their own supervisor, an interesting model from counselling, but not one adopted by the author.

(B) Lilley, David, and Hinson (2007) also describe implementing an interprofessional supervision pilot project in a hospice. They identified supervision as a key element of staff support. They commenced with individual supervision and then introduced group supervision. The group supervision finished at the end of the project although it is not clear why. One conclusion was that the different disciplines had the added benefit of learning about each others' roles, responsibility, and working styles. They were clear that reflection on practice had added benefit.

Discussion

In the author's example of establishing an inclusive programme of supervision, referred to earlier in the text, the clinical supervision was available to all members of the multi-professional team, and thus supervisors were drawn from different professions: this is seen by participants to be a strength. (Some members of the multi-professional team continue to have external supervision.) The supervisees were all allocated to groups which were not supervised by their line managers. Each group has a maximum of five members, and two trained supervisors are currently not being used because of other pressures on their time. One of the hardest tasks was to decide on groups and supervisors were given the final say. A supervision record has been developed and there are regular meetings for supervisors.

Reviewing the clinical supervision arrangements is key, and in the author's project the questionnaire developed can be used again to measure progress.

In the other two examples the supervision arrangements were made by nursing and educationalists and all had the support of their organizations.

Conclusions

The suspicions nurses have had about clinical supervision can also be found in other professions. This has probably led to the ambivalence about arranging this kind of support (Clulow, 1994). He suggested that fear of being over-managed or being 'nannied' led to people paying lip-service to supervision. It needs supervisees to be committed. Other professions, particularly social and therapeutic care, have moved towards embracing supervision. Organizations such as hospices and palliative care teams struggle to manage the needs of the patients, the organization, and the workers (Olney, 2001). There is anecdotal evidence and some research that suggests that clinical supervision helps.

The need to value staff and to keep them emotionally safe is generally recognized as being important in specialist palliative care because of the work done in identifying workforce stress and burnout. Generally it is acknowledged that working with death and dying on a daily basis is tough. The intensity of the often brief helping relationship means that behaviour can be misinterpreted and decision-making affected. The work needs resilient staff who can remain in touch with the emotional needs of patients and their families and be aware of their own feelings.

The problems faced by those wanting to arrange for staff supervision in any setting is highlighted in palliative care by the lack of research. In the current economic climate there is a need to focus our efforts more appropriately. Scarcity of resources often leads to projects such as those described being cut. The supervision model of separating out line management from supervision is the dominant model, but it must not undermine the manager's role. Olney (2001) points out the potential for 'splitting'. Supervision of the supervisors is the common way of regulating this.

Therefore all supervision must be contracted, whether internally or externally, and keeping notes which are shared with the group is the most open and empowered way to proceed. Can supervision be mandatory? Probably not; if supervisees are made to attend it is against the purpose of the sessions.

The focus of supervision should always be on the primary task. A 'moan session' achieves nothing. If the organization wishes to keep to task, well-facilitated clinical supervision makes a major contribution. It is about the supervisee in the work, not about personal therapy.

Finally the author believes that clinical supervision is part of staff support and good clinical governance. It allows staff to monitor themselves and to develop coping skills to stay in the work.

References

Bond, M. and Holland, S. (2001). *Skills of Clinical Supervision for Nurses*. Buckingham: Open University Press.

Bishop, V. (2007). Clinical supervision: What is it? Why do we need it? In V. Bishop (ed.), *Clinical Supervision in Practice*. Basingstoke: Palgrave.

Chilvers, R. (2009). Implementing a clinical supervision programme for nurses in a hospice setting. *International Journal of Palliative Care Nursing*, **15**(12), 615–19.

Clulow, C. (1994). Balancing care and control: The supervisory relationship as a focus for promoting organisational health. In A. Obholzer and V.Z. Roberts (eds), *The Unconscious At Work*. London: Routledge.

Edwards, D., et al. (2005). Factors influencing the effectiveness of clinical supervision. *Journal of Psychiatric and Mental Health Nursing*, **12**, 405–14.

Faugier, J. (1996). Clinical supervision and mental health nursing. In T. Sandford and K. Gournay (eds), *Perspectives in Mental Health Nursing*. London: Balliere Tindall.

Firth, P. (2005). Groupwork in palliative care. In P. Firth, G. Luff, and D. Oliviere (eds), *Loss, Change and Bereavement in Palliative Care*. Maidenhead: Open University Press.

Firth, P. (2006). Patients and their families. In F. Stiefel (ed.), *Communication in Cancer Care*. Heidelberg: Springer.

Fletcher, S. (2008). Supervision needs of nurses working in the community. *International Journal of Palliative Care Nursing*, **14**(4), 196–200.

Freshwater, D. (2007). Reflective practice and clinical supervision: Two sides of the same coin. In V. Bishop (ed.), *Clinical Supervision in Practice*. Basingstoke: Palgrave.

Hawkins, P. and Shoet, R. (2000). *Supervision in the Helping Professions*. Milton Keynes: Open University Press.

Hyrkas, K. (2005). Clinical supervision, burnout and job satisfaction among mental health and psychiatric nurses in Finland. *Issues in Mental Health Nursing*, **26**, 531–56.

Johns, C. (1994). Guided reflection. In A. Palmer, S. Burns, and C. Bulman (eds), *Reflective Practice in Nursing: The Growth of the Professional Practitioner*. Oxford: Blackwell Science.

Kadushin, A. (1992). *Supervision in Social Work*, 3rd edn. New York: Columbia University Press.

Kelly, B., et al. (2001). A survey of community mental health nurses: Perceptions of clinical supervision in Northern Ireland. *Journal of Psychiatric and Mental Health Nursing*, **1**, 33–44.

Lilley, L., David, M., and Hinson, P. (2007). Implementing inter-professional supervision within a hospice setting. *Cancer Nursing Practice*, **6**(2), 20–5.

McCloskey, S. and Taggart, L. (2010). How much compassion have I left? An exploration of occasional stress among children's palliative care nurses. *International Journal of Palliative Care Nursing*, **6**(5), 233–40.

Olney, F. (2001). Management, supervision and practice. *Professional Social Work*, May.

Proctor, B. (1988). *Supervision: A Working Alliance* (video training material). St Leonards-on-Sea: Alexia Publications.

Reith, M. and Payne, M. (2009). *Social Work in End-of-life and Palliative Care*. Bristol: The Policy Press.

Tuckman, B.V. (1965). Development sequence in small groups. *Psychological Bulletin*, **4**, 274–84.

Chapter 14

When answers elude us: spiritual care as a tool for healing

Rena Arshinoff

Professionals who work in the field of healthcare today face overwhelming challenges. Offering oneself to care for individuals who are ill and suffering in a work environment that is often fast-paced can be exhausting with high acuity level patients and work hours that are long. While healthcare workers bring dedication and caring to their work, compassion fatigue and burnout are occupational hazards under such circumstances, especially for nurses. Working in a multidisciplinary team helps professionals know there is support from colleagues, usually in the form of sharing clinical responsibilities and formulating a plan of care that outlines goals for patients. The bigger challenge lies in ensuring that they receive the spiritual support they need for themselves to remain healthy, thrive in their chosen work, and remember why they do the difficult work that they do.

Kash et al. (2000, p. 1633) observed that health professionals who care for dying patients or those with terminal illnesses are at increased risk of emotional exhaustion and decreased empathy in comparison with those working in general medicine (Kearney et al., 2009, p. 1156). Kearney et al. explain that oncologists and oncology staff often develop long-standing relationships with patients over time and become hopeful that treatment will offer more time to them. When their patients become sicker and die of their illness, they are personally upset and grieve for their patients who they have come to know (Kearney et al., p. 1156).

Spiritual care for health professionals takes a variety of forms. While some health-care workers seek out personal advice, many, if not most, do not. Spiritual support is not synonymous with religious support; spirituality entails searching for meaning in the work they do and the significant role they play in the lives of their patients. To this end, spiritual support to health professionals often occurs in less direct ways and might seem camouflaged in the provision of spiritual care to their patients instead. This chapter highlights some particular issues for staff presented by patients by means of case studies that address specific spiritual issues; support of staff with examples drawn from my own clinical areas as a chaplain; the provision of opportunities for nurses to reflect in reflection groups; and the use of Biblical texts in spiritual care.

Caring for the ill: a spiritual profession

While health often refers to one's physical state, a holistic approach also includes emotional and spiritual components. Like physical illness, emotional and/or spiritual ailments can seriously affect an individual's ability to function. Caregivers give a great deal to their patients, often working in high stress areas with many ill people at a given time. Compassion fatigue is an occupational hazard as they run the risk of over-extending themselves partially due to the pressures put on them by the healthcare system and partially due to insufficient self-care. Sometimes they wonder about the 'fairness' of life as they bear witness to human suffering. To care for the ill brings healthcare workers face to face with monumental questions of their own as they watch some of their biggest fears played out before them in their patients and their families. Fundamental beliefs and spiritual tenets can be challenged in even the most experienced health professional.

Finding meaning in our life and in what we do is a spiritual quest for each individual. Spirituality, in contrast to religion, is broad and personal and involves a relationship with what we call the transcendent, something bigger than ourselves. For some of us, that means God, whereas others feel more of a connection with nature, community, animals, a cause, or anything that holds unique significance to them as part of the larger world. Spirituality does not own a specific dogma or set of religious rites, although this may certainly be a component of one's unique spirituality. We all search to find meaning in our lives as we live out what holds importance for us. Zerwekh writes that everyone has a spirit or is spiritual whether or not they consider themselves to be religious (Zerwekh, 2008, p.215). When our personal belief system in which we find comfort and peace is threatened, we may experience a spiritual crisis. In watching their patients suffer, caregivers are frequently called to question the randomness of what seems unfair and find themselves searching for purpose in what they do. Abraham Joshua Heschel, a Jewish philosopher of the twentieth century, said it is vital for doctors, nurses, and other health professionals to search and ask themselves what illness does not only to their patients but also to themselves as they ask why good people are afflicted with diseases that may not be curable, cause disability, or break families apart in their turmoil (Puchalski, 2006, p. 104). Florence Nightingale said that making life better for another person or providing awareness or knowledge were expressions of spirituality and a way of connecting with God (Burkhardt and Nagai-Jacobson, 2002, p. 7).

The pressures of working in healthcare

Those who work in healthcare settings today are faced with the realities of the intense acuity of their patients, heavy workloads, and high turnover of colleagues who experience both physical and spiritual exhaustion in their work. Provision of spiritual care for healthcare workers offers potential for relieving some of the burden and adding new insight into the experience of illness and providing care. None of us is immune to our own ultimate death and to the potential of falling ill; moreover, we are each vulnerable to those feelings we prefer to ignore. Despite this, healthcare workers must move from one patient to the next, fulfilling clinical goals of treatment; failing to complete such goals or watching patients succumb to their illness is oftentimes seen today by health professionals as failure of treatment. Worsening illness is to be avoided at all costs and death as a natural event has lost its place in the natural cycle of life. The notion of death as a holy event is difficult to fathom for professionals whose mandate it is to heal. Yet spiritual healing is possible even when physical cure does not occur. Health professionals are in a challenging position to realize this as well as to care for themselves in a holistic way, if they are in turn to provide such care to their patients, especially on units of cumulative loss.

The role of the chaplain

Chaplains play a unique role in supporting health professionals who struggle with questions concerning the fairness of life, why good people suffer, and the always present query 'why me?', to which there are no clear answers. Nurses are highly skilled professionals trained to provide care that involves meticulous precision and knowledge. They care deeply for those in their charge and are a major component of their healing journey. Many health professionals feel challenged when their patients present them with big existential questions. Nurses in particular face such a situation and many have told me it is easier to provide physical care than listening to their patients express their feelings; they often feel vulnerable themselves. Physiotherapists, occupational therapists, and speech language pathologists teach individuals to relearn skills they once had. Now vulnerable, they share their deepest fears and worries with professionals who may feel ill equipped for such conversations. After years of training to become clinical practitioners, health professionals believe they should be able to handle such situations, but when challenged are often reticent to ask for help; isolation in one's job as a result is not uncommon. The build-up of such situations along with heavy workloads and physical fatigue can lend itself to compassion fatigue and ultimate burnout. As a new chaplain, I naively expected members of the team to reach out and almost 'line up' for personal counselling; however, I learned that it was up to me to be creative in providing such opportunities by thinking of how health professionals might break the barrier of seeking support for themselves.

Reflection groups

Nurses work hard in meeting the needs of their patients regarding both technical tasks and the laying on of hands, often with a number of patients at a given time and requiring flexibility and organization. They are frequently exhausted, feeling run down and not appreciated by their institution. Nurses' reflection groups offer the opportunity to feel acknowledged and valued. I have conducted such groups during a specific time set aside and designated as 'inservice'. During these groups, we have talked about what it is like to work on their specific hospital unit, have had readings, reflections, meditation, and discussion.

One of the units on which I conducted such a group specializes in head and neck cancer. I asked the nurses how it felt to work with patients who had disfiguring surgery. Many spoke of this difficulty and some even expressed their fear of how they would be able to handle it if they or a loved one had to endure such difficulty. One nurse honestly said that he preferred to go into the patient's room if he had to provide medication, check the intravenous, or do a procedure. If however, the patient wanted to talk about how he/she looks or the future, this nurse felt very threatened. He preferred to call the chaplain to deal with this instead. This honesty enabled us to speak about what emotions these patients elicited in them and why it is difficult to face the real situation of looking 'grotesque', as one patient put it. We talked about how our identity is so caught up in how we look and even touched on the notion of being created in God's image. As a group we pondered the question: do these patients still reflect the notion of God's image, whatever that may be for each individual? This is a profound spiritual question as these nurses strive to provide excellent and holistic healthcare to patients who look frightening. The group provided safety and honesty.

During each of these sessions I invite each nurse to choose from a variety of shells that I bring. I choose shells because they once had life in them. This is the impetus for our discussion about their patients and their struggle with illness and death. I ask them to hold the shell while we have a guided meditation and focus on what the shell symbolizes for them. Meditation with soothing music and time for reflection following such discussions allows for a short escape from the demanding workload as they each reflect on their own spiritual needs and healing.

The grief of health professionals

Caregivers are often reserved about discussing how they feel when their patients die, especially in a group setting. Reflection groups do not necessarily lend themselves to such exploration of emotions. I placed a lovely journal in the lounge on one unit with the name of a patient who had died on each page and invited the nurses to write a sentence or two about their relationship with that person. There was no requirement to sign their name. To my dismay, only one nurse entered a statement into this journal; handwriting is recognizable. Try as I may, I have learned that the best way to discuss patients who died is to do so one on one; nurses tend to keep their emotions to themselves in an attempt to maintain their professional persona.

Many hospitals today conduct memorial services to remember individuals who have died. Families and staff are invited to attend but few healthcare workers attend such services. While they feel the pain of loss when their patients die, nurses, social workers, and their colleagues rarely grieve in such an open forum and in ways that are so public. Some may attend a funeral of a patient they came to know well, but grieving if done at all, generally occurs in a more private way. I have also come to learn that nurses often grieve their patients in a way that demonstrates what they do best: by advocating for their patients. This is most evident in ways that reflect their professional role, that is, by attending Mortality Rounds and explaining what had happened for their patients if they feel a poor judgement was made, or reflecting on how well the patient had done until a certain point; specific interactions with family members; being a part of the advanced directives or living will; or how they provided a specific type of care. Once these topics are established, nurses feel free to discuss their patient and 'grieve' in the context of the nursing care they provided, or following doctors' orders concerning which they have had mixed feelings. Emotions of anger and sadness are sometimes elicited during Mortality Rounds but they are well within the realm of professional conduct, clearly reflecting the general attitude nurses have of not demonstrating much emotion about their patients. Attending these meetings is, for nurses, an important forum for grieving. I often observe extended discussion about their patients even after the Mortality Rounds meeting has formally concluded.

To care for the dying

To care for the dying is both powerful and difficult work. Neimeyer writes that health-care specialists who have a high level of death anxiety use more avoidance coping behaviour as a way of coping with their own fear of death (Braun, 2010, p. E47). A number of studies conducted primarily among oncology nurses seek to understand their attitudes toward death and how these impact care. Wong et al. (1994, p. 121) outlined three components of death acceptance: neutral acceptance in which death is recognized as a natural part of life that will happen to everyone; approach acceptance in which death is perceived as a stepping stone to a better afterlife (this has been found to be associated with a higher degree of religious observance); and escape acceptance in which death is perceived as an escape from a life of pain and suffering (Braun, 2010, p. E44). A current study by Braun found that more religious nurses had a significant relationship with both approach acceptance and escape acceptance. Nurses who reported a higher fear of death and had more death avoidance were less positive about caring for dying patients. It was also found that older nurses tended to be less likely to exhibit death avoidance (Braun, 2010, p. E46). In their seminal study of 403 nurses, Rooda et al. concluded that nurses' personal feelings influence how they cope with caring for dying patients; these feelings are comprised of determinants of cultural, societal, philosophical, religious, personal, and cognitive frameworks (Rooda et al., 1999, p. 1683). Changes can occur over time with new experiences. Such findings indicate that nursing education requires training in the care of dying patients and their families as well as the need for continued support to nurses who care for dying individuals; moreover, spiritual support must be an integral component of ongoing education that hospitals provide for their staff.

The goal of providing support to healthcare workers, and particularly nurses, who choose not to talk about the death of their patients, is indeed challenging. Perry observed that identifying similarities between themselves and a patient with respect to age or family circumstance allows nurses to appreciate how that patient wants to be treated. This in turn allows for a high level of trust in the nurse by the patient, and the nurse feels connection with that individual (Perry, 2008, p. 87). This provides a realization that the patient is a person with a name, a family, and a set of characteristics unrelated to the medical diagnosis alone.

I recently worked with nurses who cared for a young woman in her twenties who died of cancer shortly after her diagnosis. Many of the nurses who cared for her are very close in age. She died soon after discharge from the hospital and many of the nurses were compelled to talk about how she died, their role in caring for her, and the family dynamics they encountered among her family members. Using the power of narrative as a tool for grieving, I spoke individually with many of them who appreciated the opportunity to remember this patient, who represented not only someone for whom they provided nursing care, but also whose courage represented their own fears. Narrative knowledge helps people understand the meaning and significance of stories as it provides a meaningful comprehension of a situation to the person who is doing the telling (Charon, 2001, p. 1898). Charon writes that this practice helps practitioners to identify and interpret their own emotional responses to their patients, to make sense of their own life journeys, and to face sick and dying patients (Charon, 2001, p. 1899).

This is a powerful tool for supporting healthcare workers as they deal with very critically ill patients who bring them face to face with personal spiritual challenges.

Spiritual support to health professionals by the chaplain as a team member

Nurses' attitudes toward chaplains and spiritual care vary from one unit to another. In my experience in big trauma and medical centres, my presence on most units is much appreciated. In addition to direct contact with patients, as a member of a multidisciplinary team, I attend medical rounds almost daily in order to serve as an important link and a further means of providing spiritual care in a holistic sense. This allows healthcare workers to appreciate the presence and the contribution of spiritual care to the well-being of their patients and to themselves. Not only nurses but physiotherapists, dieticians, and social workers make referrals for their patients and for themselves as well. Physicians often look to the chaplain for support in the need of breaking bad news to families and sometimes to share their own feelings around difficult or emotional cases. Sometimes there is the need to have an insight that is not covered in the medical textbooks, as illustrated in the following two case studies.

Sonia

Sonia was an 85-year-old widowed Jewish woman suffering from cardiac failure and had experienced a number of transient ischemic attacks. She was closely monitored in a level 2 intensive care unit. Sonia had two children—a daughter and her husband who were observant Orthodox Jews, and a son and his wife who practised Conservative Judaism. She had a poor prognosis and was showing signs of no longer responding to treatment. At a family meeting requested by the medical team to discuss the relevant issues, Sonia's children differed in their views about their mother's care. Whereas her son understood the implications of resuscitation, compression, and intubation in the event of a cardiac arrest, her daughter was unable to reconcile herself to the fact that the doctors were proposing a 'do not resuscitate' plan for her mother. Furthermore, the most serious decision for Sonia's daughter concerned that of feeding. Sonia, a Holocaust survivor, had a feeding tube, and her daughter insisted that a palliative status was cruel for her mother, who had been starved in her early years and always wanted to live. She could not bring herself to withhold feeds because she likened this to murder.

Judaism holds life as tantamount above all. Life is to be considered at all times and basic requirements such as nutrition and fluids are not to be withheld. Moreover, once a treatment has been started, it is not be withdrawn. At the same time, Judaism teaches that we are forbidden to prolong death, especially if the individual is suffering. The ethical challenge that arises is complex: where is the fine line that demarcates prolonging life from prolonging death? The attending physician and the nurses were very concerned about Sonia, who was clearly suffering, and her daughter, who could not make an informed decision until this meeting. A critical component of this family meeting took place when I discussed Jewish legal issues alongside the doctor and team members who presented the medical information to her children. Sonia's daughter was relieved when she learned that palliative care status did not imply that her mother would be denied feeds. The healthcare team was appreciative of the role of the chaplain to provide this component of care as it relieved them of the frustration of not understanding why this family had difficulty with their decision for treatment until it was discussed within a Jewish context.

Joan

Members of the healthcare team may find themselves working with patients and families who have difficulty in decision-making over circumstances that are threatening to their well-being. While the situation may appear to have an obvious solution to the healthcare workers, the decision may not be so easy for the individual. An example of such a situation was Joan, who was diabetic and presented with a gangrenous toe. Over time, her situation worsened, resulting in the amputation of the toe. Shortly thereafter, the gangrene spread to cover one-third of her foot. The need for amputation was obvious to all the staff caring for her, but her family hoped to find alternative treatments that could save the leg. Her pain was intense and she was no longer able to endure physiotherapy. The dietician attempted to establish a diet for her that would meet her diabetic needs as well as the requirement for increased protein for healing. The social worker could not begin to consider discharge planning because there was no clear treatment plan in place that would determine discharge requirements. The medical specialists came day after day only to learn that no decision had been made. The most intense anger was experienced by the nursing staff. Each of the nurses who cared for Joan was frustrated by the situation and found it increasingly difficult to care for this individual and her family who could not make a decision about a situation that seemed so clear cut. Furthermore, Joan was occupying a hospital bed that the staff felt could be used to allow another person to have the treatment he/she needed.

As the chaplain on the unit, I met with Joan and her family to support them in the difficult decision that faced them. Joan was the most receptive to amputation, recognizing that she needed to move forward with getting her life in order by having the pain resolved and starting anew with a prosthesis. It took many counselling sessions with this family until they made the decision for amputation. They also needed support and help in making meaning of the difficult situation before them and for Joan to find a new wholeness in the changed body she would have. She and her family searched, cried, and asked where God was for them until the decision was finalized. Following surgery, she looked forward to planning for her prosthesis and a new beginning. During the time that I worked with them, the multi-disciplinary team patiently waited for the choice this family would make. My involvement with this family allowed the nurses to move away from the intensity of their emotions and to hear from me about the fears experienced by this family. When the surgery finally took place, the nursing staff expressed their extreme appreciation for the support they received by my involvement. Working with a family such as Joan's brought everyone face to face with the horror of amputation and the concern that the gangrene could spread during the delay while the decision was being made. Nurses were challenged by the extended period of time the family needed and they were placed in a situation in which they needed to become aware that this represented a spiritual crisis for this family.

Joan's family presented a new scenario for the nurses because most patients they care for have already made the decision for amputation prior to admission; in this case, Joan's foot worsened while she was in hospital and the medical requirements changed for her. These nurses were placed in a situation in which their clinical skills were put on hold and they had to examine their personal fears and spiritual questions represented by Joan's situation. Despite this, the nurses were guarded in discussing their own fears. The entire team was pleased when Joan made her decision and they were able to provide excellent care to her. As discussed earlier, the clinical care nurses provide can be easier for them to work with than the emotional chaos some patients undergo. Certainly some nurses were more comfortable than others in supporting Joan through this difficult time. The provision of spiritual care to Joan and her family was pivotal in helping to facilitate discussion and make the ultimate decision; moreover, it took some pressure off the nurses. In this way, spiritual care imparted by the chaplain provided important support to the health professionals in a non-direct way.

Suffering: the unique experiences of healthcare workers

Regardless of the type of unit caregivers work on, they experience conflict when their own belief system is confronted with providing care to their patients that may prolong suffering or that is medically futile. Nurses especially sometimes find themselves caught in a disagreement among members of the medical team and experience moral distress as they attempt to provide the best care possible to their patients while maintaining a professional position with their colleagues (Ferrell and Coyle, 2008, p. 93). This is often experienced in a big acute care and trauma centre. I recently met a nurse in the hospital lobby leaving his shift in the early morning, looking despondent. He explained that he was assigned to a very difficult case: a young person who was the victim of a tragic car accident brought to the high-level intensive care unit and dying; the driver of the other car, who was responsible for the accident, suffered only minor injuries. He struggled as he found himself resentful of that 'unfairness'. Nurses and healthcare workers can find themselves in a position of judgement when such events occur. Like this nurse, they may also experience ambivalent feelings when their patient is the perpetrator and such feelings need to be acknowledged and worked with.

He mentioned that he saw himself in this individual close to his own age, with young children as his own. He wondered if he had provided good nursing care; his own competency came into question as he reflected on the unfairness of this painful situation. I shared with him what my own observations of him as a nurse have been and the excellent care I have watched him give to critically ill and dying patients in the intensive care unit. I listened to his lament of how difficult it is to work in a trauma centre and his worry that his care may not make a difference. He commented that he was going home to hug his daughter. As we talked about what he provided to the family, he realized that his care did make a difference for them. This dialogue took place in the midst of a busy hospital lobby but it was where and when he needed it. The operational methodology of providing spiritual care is to meet the person where he or she is, physically, emotionally, and spiritually. Upon leaving each other, he said 'thank you; I needed that'.

On another day, I was paged by the manager of a high stress unit. One of her staff members on the multi-disciplinary team was in tears. She had been transferred to complete a required rotation in her unit and was having difficulty watching the suffering of so many people. Through her tears, she said that she could not cope with the relentless distress and anguish she witnessed. She was experiencing some significant changes in her personal life which she did not realize initially were affecting her ability to handle the difficulty of her clinical cases. She questioned where God was. Ferrell and Coyle write of how nurses may become silenced when confronted with providing what appears to be futile care; such silencing, they write, may lead to a loss of personhood and to stifling personal values and beliefs (Ferrell and Coyle, 2008, p. 96). This healthcare worker (not a nurse) was fortunate to work for a manager who recognized the value of spiritual support and took the initiative to call the chaplain who could provide it at the time that this individual needed it the most, immediately at that precise moment.

Rituals

Rituals help healthcare workers know they are appreciated. While health professionals try their very best to offer compassionate care to their patients, there are times when the most pressing concern is the completion of clinical tasks, sometimes resulting in barely enough time to take care of themselves during a busy shift. A significant ritual that health professionals appreciate is the blessing of the hands in which each person is acknowledged with a short blessing and the pouring of water on their hands. Water, so symbolic of life, and poured over their hands that represent the work they do in the 'laying of hands' acknowledges staff in a meaningful way by those who work with them and those for whom they work. Wofford and Yoder write that each time she does this ritual with hospital staff, the short blessing touches their spiritual core and reminds them why they chose the career they did—to offer compassion and caring to those in need (Wofford and Yoder, 2005).

As a chaplain at a large acute care hospital that also is the home for many Canadian war veterans who live there, I was often called to partake in a beautiful ritual that was initiated a number of years ago when a veteran dies. In a moving tribute to the veteran for his/her military action and sacrifice, family and nursing staff gather around the bed of the individual who has died and a Canadian flag is placed upon the body bag. The chaplain acknowledges the veteran's gift to us as a final honour. In many cases, family members are out of town, unable to attend, especially if the death occurs during the night, or if they are no longer alive. The nurses know these residents very well and those who are present on that shift attend this beautiful, dignified, and brief ceremony. I always asked the nurses present if they would like to add some of their own words about the person who has died. Without fail, they mentioned that being included in the flag ritual is a very meaningful and spiritual experience for them as they offer praise and thanks to the individual they came to know.

The use of Biblical texts: compassion fatigue in the Bible

I recently facilitated a Jewish bereavement support group in which we studied Biblical and Rabbinic texts as an adjunct to discussion. Small snippets of verses were introduced and the members of the group found these to be very helpful. The use of these texts was not for religious purposes but rather as identification with the Jewish tradition of study. Furthermore, it was clear that Biblical texts allow bereaved individuals to read stories of their ancestors who also were ordinary people who loved and lost, experienced a myriad of emotions, felt despair and abandonment, and cried out to God in anger, sadness, and fear. They too searched for meaning to their suffering. And most important of all, they found ultimate healing.

The lessons learned in Biblical texts can also help support health professionals in preventing or addressing burnout. We read about the burden Moses was under as he led the Israelites out of Egypt. Following the opposition of Pharaoh with each plague, the acquiescence to leave, gathering a huge throng of people together, and the pressure of crossing the Sea of Reeds, Moses had the task of being advisor, judge, and counsellor to all. Needless to say, this was a formidable task. Moses was burdened with the responsibility of being magistrate for the people who were now out of their familiar home in strange surroundings and terrifying circumstances; they were vulnerable and frightened.

Jethro, Moses' father-in-law, had the sensitivity, insight, and foresight needed to advise Moses, who was the leader of the 600,000 individuals as they wandered in the wilderness. Jethro recognized that Moses was suffering from bearing this burden alone. He saw the magnitude of the job entrusted to Moses and recognized that Moses could not do it alone. He gently approached Moses with advice recommending that he select capable individuals to assume leadership in partnership with him. 'Make it easier for yourself by letting them share the burden with you.' Jethro exhibited humility as he told Moses that he would give him counsel, and God would be with him. Moses, exhausted from the many demands and huge workload of his position, acknowledged the support and good advice.

Jethro had the insight to recognize that Moses would be worn out by assuming the huge job single-handedly. He said, 'you will surely wear yourself out, and these people as well. For the task is too heavy for you; you cannot do it alone' (Exodus, JPS Tanakh, 2003, p. 153). Moreover, Jethro had the foresight that if Moses assigned others to settle smaller disputes and brought larger ones to Moses, that Moses would be able to bear up; 'and all these people too will go home unwearied'. Moses did indeed listen to the advice offered by his father-in-law, recognizing the wisdom and sensitivity displayed by Jethro. Like Moses, healthcare workers need such support and to know that this support is there to be had.

Conclusion

Spirituality touches on profound and sacred aspects of people's lives (Lloyd-Williams, 2008, p. 198). This holds true for patients as well as for the health professionals who care for them. While a great deal of attention is focused on spiritual needs of patients and their families, we must not overlook the needs of healthcare workers who are challenged each day to tend to their patients, who often need to share their deepest and most profound fears, leaving some healthcare workers unprepared to support them in their suffering (Norlander, 2008, p. 52). We help health professionals best by letting them know there are spiritual care providers on the multi-disciplinary team trained in this area, and we can help by providing spiritual care for them in the role they play in caring for others. If we help them in the search for meaning in the work they do, they can thrive in making a difference for others. Provision of spiritual care to health professionals offers a key contribution to healing, connection, and self-growth and facilitates recognition of the holiness of life even when answers to painful questions elude us.

References

Braun, M., Gordon, D., and Uziely, B. (2010). Associations between oncology nurses' attitudes toward death and caring for dying patients. *Oncology Nursing Forum*, **37**(1), 43–9.

Burkhardt, M.A. and Nagai-Jacobson, M.G. (2002). *Spirituality: Living Our Connectedness*. Albany, NY: Delmar.

Charon, R. (2001). Narrative medicine: A model for empathy, reflection, profession, and trust. *Journal of the American Medical Association*, **286**(15), 1897–1901.

Exodus 18:22. *JPS Hebrew–English Tanakh* (2003). Philadelphia: Jewish Publishing Society.

Ferrell, B.R. and Coyle, N. (2008). *The Nature of Suffering and the Goals of Nursing*. New York: Oxford University Press.

Kash, K.M., Holland, J.C., Breitbart, W., *et al.* (2000). Stress and burnout in oncology. *Oncology*, **14**(11), 1621–37.

Kearney, M., Weininger, A.B., Vachon, M.L.S., Harrison, R.L., and Mount, B.M. (2009). Self-care of physicians caring for patients at the end of life. *Journal of the American Medical Association*, **301**(11), 1155–64.

Lloyd-Williams, M. (2008). *Psychosocial Issues in Palliative Care*. Oxford: Oxford University Press.

Norlander, L. (2008). *To Comfort Always*. Indianapolis, IN: Sigma Theta Tau International.

Perry, B. (2008). Why exemplary oncology nurses seem to avoid compassion fatigue. *Canadian Oncology Nursing Journal*, **18**(2), 87–92.

Puchalski, C.M. (2006). *A Time for Listening and Caring*. New York: Oxford University Press.

Rooda, L.A., Clements, R., and Jordan, M.L. (1999). Research briefs: Nurses' attitudes towards death and caring for dying patients. *Oncology Nursing Forum*, **26**(10), 1683–7.

Wofford, S.R. and Yoder Jr, J. (2005). Blessing of the hands: A gift to the staff. *PlainViews: An e-letter for Chaplains and Other Healthcare Providers*, **2**(4).

Wong, P., Reker, G., and Gesser, G. (1994). Death Attitude Profile—Revised: A multidimensional measure of attitudes toward death. In R.A. Neimeyer (ed.), *Death Anxiety Handbook: Research, Instrumentation, and Application*. Washington DC: Taylor and Francis, 121–48.

Zerwekh, J.V. (2008). *Nursing Care at the End of Life: Palliative Care for Patients and Families*. Philadelphia: F.A. Davis Company.

Chapter 15

Reflections on caring: a brief essay on presence

Ted Bowman

In the pages that follow, a lifetime of work as a grief and family educator will be scrutinized and reflected upon for thoughts, recommendations, and resources about the nature and importance of presence when engaging in caring. A rationale for this singular focus will be provided. To accomplish this, two filters will be utilized. Poetry therapy or bibliotherapy is the creative use of literary sources, writing, and storytelling for therapeutic purposes. Like its siblings—drama, art, music, and dance therapy—it is seen as a legitimate tool that complements other therapeutic and caring processes. In this case, stories can and will enrich these reflections about caring. In addition, the framework of the ethical-spiritual will be used. The ethical spiritual will (see Baines, 2002) is a statement of learnings about life. Especially appropriate as part of life-review (see Butler, 1974), an ethical-spiritual will can be a statement or testimony about any insights and wisdom gained through experiences over a lifespan or about particular moments or components of life. When I began to write this chapter, I steadily found my thoughts and examples as a grief and family educator converging around the crucial dimension of presence and attendance in the caring exchange. These pages, therefore, can be thought of as a reflective statement by an educator and trainer of carers/helpers about what he believes to be the essential dimension for caring.

The medicine of friendship

Asked to recall the most frequent question when training carers in hospice, hospital, bereavement, mental health, and related settings, my response is quick, clear, and without doubt. 'What do you say to someone who is suffering?' That question, more than any other, seems to be a source of curiosity and anxiety for many carers. Caring professionals and volunteers want to say or do something that lifts spirits, makes a difference, alleviates suffering, lightens a load, or is beneficial. When pressed, one hears that just being present in the face of suffering is the core desire and value. What to say has less to do with the actual words and more to do with how to be fully there with another who is hurting. I'm convinced that competence with tools of communication, medical or mental health techniques, and creative intervention strategies must be inextricably intertwined with the experience of presence emanating from the service provider or carer. Further, attention to compassion fatigue, burnout, caring teamwork, and ethics and boundaries must be linked with assistance in responses to a

seemingly universal cry of carers, 'What do you say or do in the face of suffering people?' Even specific queries, such as how to respond to an angry caregiver or patient,
include how to be present with someone that might be scary, intimidating, or off-
putting. Papadatou places presence at the centre of what she described as the accompanying process (Papadatou, 2009). Kearney calls it companioning (Kearney, 2000).
Here are other metaphors and images from memoirs and the helping literature.

> 'Barbara, we've known each other for well over a year, and we've been honest with each
> other every step of the way.'
>   Briefly, her lips trembled, and then she regained her composure. Her eyes told me she
> knew what I was about to say.
>   'I know of no medicines that I can give at this point to help you.' . . .
>   Barbara shook her head. 'No . . . ' she said. 'You do have something to give. You have
> the medicine of friendship.' (Groopman, 2004)

Oncologist Jerome Groopman wrote about this experience, stating it was a profound
teaching moment that shaped the rest of his medical career. He emphasized that he did
not learn about the medicine of friendship in medical school classes, residences, or from
esteemed colleagues. Rather, as is often the case for those willing to take note of a range
of teachers, he learned about it from a patient. It was a caring intersection: the oncologist
cared for his patient; the patient yearned for companionship even when medical services
were limited. She called it the medicine of friendship; he responded with presence.

Bereft father Nicholas Wolterstorff, following the accidental death of his son,
wrote:

> If you think your task as comforter is to tell me that really, all things considered, it's not so
> bad, you do not sit with me in my grief but place yourself off in the distance away from
> me. Over there, you are of no help . . . To comfort me, you have to come close. Come sit
> beside me on my mourning bench. (Wolterstorff, 1987)

This father, like Barbara, seems to be describing something more than technique or
skill. The psychiatrist and trainer of psychotherapists Peter Lomas provocatively
asserted there is danger in teaching or seeking techniques for carers. 'The limitation of
technique is at no time more apparent than when the therapist is faced with naked
grief, when someone is crying helplessly in the grip of an experience that is too painful
for words, when the therapist can say nothing that would not seem presumptuous or
trivial' (Lomas, 1999). Wolterstorff's plea—come sit—comes after an overview of
many of the verbal responses to him and his family following the death of their son.
He described some verbal responses as wonderful, others not. But, as a grieving father,
he declared that the heart speaks more loudly than the words spoken. He echoed
Lomas's comments about technique. Even not-so-good words can be softened and
countered by congruent presence. Acknowledgement and validation don't necessarily
require complete accuracy to be powerfully experienced.

Kay Redfield Jamison, writing about her struggles with manic-depressive illness,
further elaborated on what to say. She described one of her carers, a psychiatrist, and
his caring capacity: 'I remember sitting in his office a hundred times during those grim
months and each time thinking, What on earth can he say that will make me feel better
or keep me alive?' Then, she went on to write: 'Well, there was never anything he could

say, that's the funny thing. It was all the stupid, desperately optimistic, condescending things he didn't say that kept me alive; all the compassion and warmth I felt from him that could not have been said; all the intelligence, competence, and time he put into it; and his granite belief that mine was a life worth living' (Jamison, 1995).

Still another account: a terminally ill patient commented on what he wished from his medical provider:

> To the typical physician, my illness is a routine incident in his rounds, while for me it's the crisis of my life. I would feel better if I had a doctor who at least perceived this incongruity . . . I see no reason or need for my doctor to love me—nor would I expect him to suffer with me. I wouldn't demand a lot of my doctor's time: I just wish he would brood on my situation for perhaps five minutes, that he would give me his whole mind just once, be bonded with me for a brief space, survey my soul as well as my flesh, to get at my illness, for each man is ill in his own way. (Broyard, 1992)

As an experienced educator, I am constantly reminded that my lifetime of experiences is my rock and my quicksand. I have learned much that is valuable and enhances my competence. That experience, on the other hand, can cause me to be callous, indifferent to stories similar to many heard before. Presence in the here and now can get compromised with the there and then of previous encounters.

Dale Larson, also a teacher of carers, has named some of the essential qualities for carers in his book *The Helper's Journey*. Human presence is at the top of his list of qualities (Larson, 1993). Drawing on research, which he admitted is limited but growing, Larson indicated that the ability to be present can reduce threat and provide comfort. Larson's assertion has been supported by Papadatou. She personalized the concept when she wrote that months or years after an experience of presence, we may forget the name of the person and the details, yet recall a look, a gesture, a shared silence, a particular intonation, or a caring act that created a deep connection (Papadatou, 2009). It is important to emphasize are that her examples include both momentary and lengthy relational experiences.

The medical sociologist Arthur Frank's memoir of his heart attack and cancer experiences, *At the Will of the Body*, contain still more commentary about presence. He describs a physician providing him with a medical answer that was, as he put it, not my answer. 'I did not know . . . what I wanted the physician to say . . . But I needed some recognition of what was happening to me.' He then describes the difference between what was said and what was desired as involving the difference between disease and illness (Frank, 1991). It is, Kenneth Hardy attests, one thing to lose something that was important; it is far worse when no one in your universe recognizes that you lost it (Hardy, 2005). The failure to acknowledge another's loss is to deny that person's humanity; it is the opposite of presence. Illness, more than disease, can mean loss of innocence, loss of the future, a shattering of assumptions (see Becker, 1997; Bowman, 1994; and Janoff-Bulman, 1992).

Storm homes for carers

The American humorist Garrison Keillor, during a 'Prairie Home Companion' radio monologue, used the provocative imagery of a *storm home* to describe the wondrous power of support. He told the story of school children from the countryside being assigned an in-town storm home to which they would go should there be a snowstorm that would prevent the buses from returning them home. In his inimitable style, Keillor described the supportive power of knowing that there was someone in town ready and waiting to take care of him in an emergency. Even though he never utilized the assigned resource, the boy in the story imagined himself surrounded by caring people, just waiting to extend their hospitality to him. Hot chocolate, games, and a welcoming environment were parts of his picture of what awaited his arrival (Keillor, 1985).

My wife and I walked out of a care facility one evening with a woman friend whose husband was dying of a brain tumour. As we exited together, I asked her if there was any other way than sitting with the two of them that I/we could be helpful. She looked suspicious and asked, 'Do you really mean it?' Many people had told her that if she needed something, they would be there for her. But she reported that too many rarely came around to check or reaffirm their supportive inquiry. Assuring her that the offer was genuine, she asked me if we would clean up her house. Surprised, I asked her to say more. She said, 'Ted, it is so hard to be here in this place of dying and death everyday. I just don't have the energy to clean the house any more.' I immediately came to the conviction that if anyone needs a nurturing environment (a storm home) to come home to, it must be those who have loved ones in hospitals, hospices, and nursing homes. We cleaned her house.

'Craig crawled into bed with his wife, Alice, who was dying at the hospice. They slept together through the night. At the team meeting the next morning, the clinical director, upon reflecting on the experience, said, "That's what we aim for. We'll give the medications, change the diapers, watch the swelling, take the vitals so that a mate can be a mate instead of a practical nurse, which is what Craig would have had to be if Alice had stayed at home"' (Blaine-Wallace, 2002). The hospice was a storm home away from home.

I experienced the carer equivalent of the storm home during my first visit to Martin House Children's Hospice in the north of England. When Martin House was being created almost 25 years ago, the staff begin to foster a culture whereby one and all would attend staff support sessions not only for support when needed but also because it could be the day a colleague would need support. Most impressive is that the staff support sessions have been voluntary from their beginning until now. They are not staff meetings, they are not for purposes of supervision, nor are they required. Almost perfect attendance has been the practice for 25 years. Staff at Martin House created a storm home to surround each worker as they do their important work.

The storm home imagery applies not only to patients, clients, and their families but also to providers of care. Compassion fatigue and burnout are well-known occupational hazards for providers of care. Finding a balance between compassion fatigue and compassion satisfaction (see Stamm, 1999) is crucial for the well-being of helpers and for best practice with recipients. Presence requires self-awareness. Renowned family therapist Virginia Satir asserted that the only instrument that one brings to the helping process is oneself. Therefore, the more self-aware one is the more present he/she can be in the helping exchange (Satir, 1976). Satir called this congruence: a congruent person is in touch with . . . feelings, regardless of what is there (Satir and Baldwin, 1983).

Renee Katz's recommendation about those times when professionals weep in response to suffering is to start with self-awareness and the intersections of transference and counter-transference. 'It is our belief that if we have the courage to identify and confront the totality of our responses in patient care at the end of life, we can use it to inform and enrich our work.' Presence has received less attention, she purported, because 'until recently, end-of-life [her focal area] theorists, clinicians, practitioners, and teachers have devoted greater effort to understanding and evaluating one member of the therapeutic relationship—the patient' (Katz, 2006).

The best summary I've read for this facet of presence is, I believe, from Thich Nhat Hanh.

> To me, the practice of a healer, therapist, teacher, or any helping professional should be directed towards him or herself first, because if the helper is unhappy, he or she cannot help many people. We practice enjoying the positive elements in life in order to nourish the flower in us, and we practice in order to transform the seeds of suffering in us. Otherwise, we cannot succeed in our work helping other people. (see Hahn, 1987)

Note the attention to the full continuum of self-care, from the positive elements to the seeds of suffering. Both need attention to be congruently present.

Clarity about one's work and the teeter-totter of compassion fatigue and satisfaction can be enhanced by a team and by individual acts that aid one in reflecting on one's work. Reflective writing in medical settings is becoming more commonplace. Pioneer, Rita Charon, described this emerging focus:

> The field of narrative medicine has emerged gradually from a confluence of sources—humanities and medicine, primary care medicine, contemporary narratology, and the study of effective doctor–patient relationships. A clinical cousin of literature-and-medicine and a literary cousin of relationship-centered care, narrative medicine provides health care professionals with practical wisdom in comprehending what patients endure in illness and what they themselves undergo in the care of the sick. (Charon, 2006)

A rich variety of expressions for what Charon calls narrative medicine have recently emerged. In this chapter, I have drawn on medical memoirs to compare with and complement the 'helping' literatures. The Israeli clinicians and teachers Lynne Dale Halamish and Doron Hermoni have written a practical and profound book of case studies about encounters with grief to aid readers with self-awareness and clinical issues (Halamish and Hermoni, 2007). Gillie Bolton has written extensively about reflective writing in caring settings as a tool for discernment (see Bolton, 2002). Ann Burack-Weiss assigned caregiver memoirs to inform her teaching as she taught social work students. Reading memoirs, she believed, can and will enhance the understanding of the professionals a caregiver turns to for help (Burack-Weiss, 2006). These are examples of the use of literary, writing, and reflective tools for informing and enriching the potential for presence by carers of carers, some of which can be richer when done with colleagues.

The educator Parker Palmer declared that good teaching (I would add caring work) cannot be reduced to technique; good teaching comes from the identity and integrity of the teacher (Palmer, 1998). He argued that all helpers/carers need to create communities of caring and discernment so that the person arrives (presence), not just the body of the person. Reflective writing, provocative and supportive case review sessions, and mentors that demonstrate companioning, accompanying presences, and the medicine of friendship are steps toward more consistent presence in caring.

One could argue whether presence can be taught or not. However one states their position, introducing and providing rich examples from memoir and other accounts can at a minimum raise consciousness of its importance and some of the characteristics of presence. Too quickly moving to techniques, even those supported by research, avoids the subject and the oft-voiced cries of suffering persons for presence in the midst of their struggle. On the other hand, addressing the subject as shown here enhances awareness and points toward attitudes and skills that are part of presence.

A cruse of hope

To close this chapter, consider Cruse Bereavement Care, a United Kingdom resource, primarily staffed by volunteers, offering bereavement support. I offer you a slightly adapted version of the afterword from a celebrative book about the 50 years of Cruse Bereavement Care. My words in their commemorative volume overlap with this chapter. In this case, hope and presence are linked.

Bereavement care, whatever else it is, includes hope: hope that someone will hear the cries, hope that someone will stop by, hope for a better day tomorrow, hope to get through all the decisions, hope for release, hope for hope.

When Cruse Bereavement Care first began as a neighbour-to-neighbour (widows and widowers) effort years ago, hope, in the person of the Cruse volunteer, went down a lane or road to where someone was grieving a death. It was yet another version of caring symbolized by cruses that contain ointment, salve, and medicines. In my state of Minnesota, a version of a cruse is called the Minnesota hot dish, because food is often brought to grievers in the form of a casserole. This kind of 'cruse' is common throughout the world, though the foods vary.

Whether or not a tangible substance accompanies the carer, hope arrives. Whether or not the bereft person is ready for companionship, hope arrives. Whether or not movement toward what is sometimes called healing, progress, or acceptance is achieved, hope arrives. Whether the caring person is professional or volunteer, trained or untrained, or whether the timing is right or wrong, hope arrives.

Let me be clear, I am not saying that all bereavement care is timely, appropriate, or done well. We must continue to learn, refine, and be flexible in and about bereavement care. The early pioneers of Cruse Bereavement Care had it right when they believed that what they proposed to do was sufficiently important that those who did bereavement care needed training, support, and continuing education. What I am emphasizing is that bereavement care is most often human and the attentive presence of another caring human being suggests hope, embodies hope, and lets one know that they are not alone in their grief and bereavement. What a gift!!

Bereavement care, at its best, is counter-cultural because the grief of death can be acknowledged. When that happens, hope also happens. Debates about what hope is and is not have often occurred and will occur again and again. But, bereft people often speak about the pain of abandonment, of the absence of care, and of discovering while grieving who their 'real' friends are. The cruse of quality bereavement care contains hope that offers a balm to isolation and devaluation.

It is a ministry of presence (Bowman, 2009).

References

Baines, B. (2002). *Ethical Wills: Putting Your Values on Paper.* Cambridge: Perseus Publishing.

Becker, G. (1997). *Disrupted Lives: How People Create Meaning in a Chaotic World.* Berkeley: University of California Press.

Blaine-Wallace, W. (2002). *Water in the Wastelands: The Sacrament of Shared Suffering.* Cambridge, MA: Cowley Publications.

Bolton, G. (2002). *Reflective Practice: Writing and Professional Development.* Thousand Oaks, CA: Sage.

Bowman, T. (1994). *Loss of Dreams: A Special Kind of Grief.* St. Paul, MN: Self-published booklet.

Bowman, T. (2009). A cruse of hope. In *Voices of Cruse: 1959-2009.* Richmond, UK: Cruse Bereavement Care, 184–5.

Broyard, A. (1992). *Intoxicated by My Illness.* New York: Clarkson Potter.

Butler, R.N. (1974). Successful aging and the role of the life review. *Journal of the American Geriatrics Society,* **22**, 529–35.

Burack-Weiss, A. (2006). *The Caregiver's Tale: Loss and Renewal in Memoirs of Family Life.* New York: Columbia University Press.

Charon, R. (2006). *Narrative Medicine: Honoring the Stories of Illness.* Oxford: Oxford University Press.

Frank, A.W. (1991). *At the Will of the Body: Reflections on Illness.* New York: Houghton Mifflin.

Groopman, J. (2004). *The Anatomy of Hope: How People Prevail in the Face of Illness.* New York: Random House.

Hahn, T.N. (1987). *Being Peace.* Berkeley: Parallax Press.

Halamish, L.D. and Hermoni, D. (2007). *The Weeping Willow: Encounters with Grief.* Oxford: Oxford University Press.

Hardy, K.V. and Laszloffy, T.A. (2005). *Teens Who Hurt: Clinical Interventions to Break the Cycle of Adolescent Violence.* New York: Guilford Press.

Jamison, K.R. (1995). *An Unquiet Mind: A Memoir of Moods and Madness.* New York: Alfred A. Knopf.

Janoff-Bulman, R. (1992). *Shattered Assumptions: Towards a New Psychology of Trauma.* New York: The Free Press.

Katz, R.S. (2006). When our personal selves influence our professional work. In R.S. Katz and T.A. Johnson (eds), *When Professional Weep: Emotional and Countertransference Responses in End-of-Life Care.* New York: Routledge.

Kearney, M. (2000). *A Place of Healing: Working with Suffering in Living and Dying.* Oxford: Oxford University Press.

Keillor. G. (1985). Prairie home companion. In *Lake Wobegon Days.* New York: Viking Press.

Larson, D.G. (1993). *The Helper's Journey: Working with People Facing Grief, Loss, and Life-Threatening Illness.* Champaign, IL: Research Press.

Lomas, P. (1999). *Doing Good? Psychotherapy Out of Its Depth.* Oxford: Oxford University Press.

Palmer, P.J. (1998). *The Courage to Teach.* San Francisco: Jossey-Bass.

Papadatou, D. (2009). *In the Face of Death: Professionals Who Care for the Dying and the Bereaved.* New York: Springer.

Satir, V. (1976). *Making Contact. Millbrae: Celestial Arts.* (First heard in a month-long training with Satir in 1975.)

Satir, V. and Baldwin, M. (1983). *Satir Step by Step.* Palo Alto, CA: Science and Behavior Books.

Stamm, B.H. (ed.) (1999) *Secondary Traumatic Stress: Self-Care Issues for Clinicians, Researchers, and Educators.* Lutherville, MD: Sidran Press.

Wolterstorff. N. (1987). *Lament for a Son.* Grand Rapids, MI: William B. Eerdmans.

Afterword

Dr William Lamers

The chapters in this volume provide a comprehensive overview of the pressures involved in providing care to patients with incurable end-stage illness of various sorts. What follows is a brief overview from my personal experience of caring for dying persons and their families over the past forty years.

My experience as a physician and psychiatrist influenced my decision to develop a programme that eventually became a hospice. My motivation came out of the frustration I felt at seeing a number of patients who were experiencing disabling, chronic emotional distress because of the death of a loved one that had not been handled well by physicians. Eventually physicians were asking me to see patients of theirs who were dying, often because the physician did not know what to do, especially with what was termed 'intractable' pain.

Physician attitudes toward dying and death are formed early in life or very early in medical careers. Three years ago I was teaching fourth-year medical students about dying and death. In one exercise, each student was instructed to deliver a difficult prognosis to an actor or actress who had been trained to role-play a seriously ill patient. I thought the exercise went well. After the students left, one remained in her chair, looking concerned. When I asked what was going on, she replied that she had to change her plans for residency because of this role-playing exercise. She explained that she was going to start a cardiology training programme in three months. Until this exercise she never considered the possibility that one of her patients might die. She felt she could not deal with a dying patient. I assured her that she could not escape from death in any specialty and that there would be deaths among her family members and friends.

Herman Feifel noted that medical students and physicians have a higher level of 'death anxiety' than any other professional group.

The definitive book on early hospice development, *The Medical Work of the Knights Hospitalers of St John of Jerusalem*, does not discuss caregiver stress, probably because the caregivers, an order of religious knights, were certain that their patients were soon to be with God. They even referred to their patients as 'Our Lords, the sick.' The religious fervour of these early (twelfth-century) hospice workers no doubt sustained them through stressful times. They hired physicians to diagnose and prescribe for their patients. The cohesiveness of the religious order allowed for strong mutual support among these caregivers.

Fears and myths need to be addressed before they become embedded in a patient care programme. Facts clearly presented can help staff to deal with the physical challenges of their work. Fears, myths, and personal experiences surrounding dying and death are common and probably more important for staff to verbalize. Some staff have difficulty identifying the source of their anxiety about dying and death. Those who have no personal experience with dying or deceased persons need support. More experienced staff who make home visits with new staff are supportive by their mere presence. I have also learned that driving staff to and from a home visit leads to more open discussion of concerns than usually surfaces during an office consultation.

I witnessed a variant of stress during the years I worked in a large cancer centre. Nurses, especially recent graduates, were concerned that they might contract cancer from their patients. They were fearful they might impair their reproductive potential through proximity to patients who were receiving radiation therapy. These concerns were not openly expressed, but were shared with me during the course of my weekly support sessions.

It took me a while to realize that I had a similar problem when I volunteered to work as an orderly at a polio hospital in the early 1950s. I was assigned to the respirator ward where patients with bulbar polio were kept alive in large respirators. There was no polio vaccine at the time, only painful injections of gamma globulin for those who worked on that unit. I didn't know how stressed I was because of my exposure to patients dying of an incurable disease until several nights later when I awakened from sleep, unable to move and unable to breathe. For a short while I feared I was dying. Soon I was able to start breathing and to move my extremities.

About twenty-five years ago, during a conference on spiritual issues in end-of-life care, a nurse stood and said loudly, 'When is it going to end?' Her remarks were unexpected and referred to the stress, especially her own, of receiving dying patients transported to the palliative care unit from other parts of the state. Most died in just a few days. She told of how depressing this was as staff did not know these patients. Some families were too far away to visit. As soon as one patient died, another dying patient was brought in. She said, 'The beds never got cold.' By now she was crying and repeated, 'When will this end?' This unanticipated emotional outburst stands out in my memory as this level of distress was not present in the earlier days of this same programme when patient care was limited to the local population.

Bringing patients to a palliative care unit for the last few days of their lives can be very disheartening. At its best, hospice is a community programme. Central to good hospice care is the relationship that develops among patient, family, and hospice staff.

Unless the grief of staff can be properly externalized, verbalized, communicated, and shared, enthusiasm for doing hospice work will soon lead to staff burnout.

Over time, funding became important, as did acceptance by other areas of health-care. As more programmes developed and leaders paid attention to the impact of care on patients, families, staff, and volunteers, it was common to hear the terms 'burnout' and even 'burnin'. We began to attend to the emotional and physical well-being of those who cared for hospice patients and their families. I recall clearly the time a hospice nurse took me aside and said, 'I served two tours of duty as a "MASH" [Military Advanced Surgical Hospital] nurse in Vietnam.' She said, 'I thought that was "tough" work. Choppers would bring in wounded troops at all hours, some of them close to death from wounds. We'd try to repair them; some lived and went on to hospitals.

Others died. We never got to know them. We did the best we could. But I find that hospice is much more difficult. In hospice you get to know the patients; you come to love them . . . and then they die.' The intensity of grief when a patient died served, for most staff, as an occasion to reassess their own lives. They decided not to postpone things they wanted to do. Some reported expressing more affection for loved ones.

She continued on for years as an excellent hospice/palliative care nurse. She did not draw back from relationships that she knew would result in death and which gave her a highly personal sense of loss and grief. Not every hospice worker experiences a sense of loss when a patient dies. Death may be for some what is commonly referred to as 'a blessing'.

Patients and families also experience stress during the late stages of illness. On occasion in home care hospice we saw spouses who wanted to do everything on their own, not to share any duties with volunteers. We developed the saying, 'It's impossible for one person to be everything to a patient all the time.' Some family caregivers were more reluctant than others to allow assistance from hospice volunteers. We learned from the instance of a woman who experienced a heart attack shortly after her husband returned home for hospice care. Several factors aggravated patient/family stress during end-stage disease. Physician reluctance to 'let go' and to refer to hospice was common. Late referrals were also a problem because so many things were happening at once, and so many things needed to be done. It takes time for patients and families to receive maximum benefit from hospice care.

Some patient care situations were more difficult for me than others. A paediatrician asked me to see his 9-year-old patient, the son of another paediatrician I knew. I was reluctant and asked, 'But what can I do to help him?' The referring doctor said, 'Don't worry . . . he'll take care of you.' And he was right. I was anxious because my own children were close to the same age and I kept worrying about what I'd do if one of them developed cancer. When I visited the patient he said, 'I'm all right with what's happening. Help my mother. She's having a tough time. And tell my dad to get a new photo.' He had seen the photo of his dad in the newspaper during an appearance before a congressional committee where he sought funds for juvenile cancer research. My own anxieties about dealing with a dying child changed during that interview.

When a physician specialist in radiation oncology whom I had known for many years became a hospice patient, I sat at his bedside on what proved to be his last day. He had a lot of difficulty accepting the reality that he was dying. Suddenly he reached up and grabbed me by the collar as he shouted, 'Bill, don't let me die! I've only now begun to live!' He died soon after this exhortation. Needless to say, his death affected me deeply as he was not only a patient but a fellow physician and good friend. Within an hour or two I did something I have never done before or since. I went home and went to bed in the early afternoon. Before long I was awaked from a startling dream in which I was reading in my medical school library. A sudden powerful gust of wind blew out all the windows and cleared the shelves of books. The dream, I believe, was a way of recognizing the devastation wrought by death. My friend's death reminded me of my own mortality. It was a truly stressful experience, yet it was also beneficial.

A hospice nurse asked me to make a home visit with her to a home where a young mother was dying of cancer. After I saw that all possible excellent nursing care had been provided, I returned to the hospice office. The patient died just after I left. The nurse stayed to handle all that needed to be done, then returned to the office. I watched her enter the office and walk toward her desk. Suddenly, she fell to the floor and began to sob. I went to her, as did other staff. As I tried to determine what had happened she blurted out with much emotion, 'It just struck me—what would happen to my children if I were to die!?' She had children of approximately the same ages. I was interested that this nurse had not grasped the way she identified with this patient until after the patient died.

There is no way to prevent staff from identifying with their patients, especially those that remind them of loved ones. Other staff will experience increased stress with certain types of patients. Stress cannot always be prevented, but careful programme planning that includes attention to the selection, training, supervision, and support of staff is essential. The major source of distress in hospice care derives from poor programme planning and inadequate attention to staff needs.

Caring for dying persons often results in changes in staff beliefs and assumptions about life and death. In most instances this results in the development of improved interpersonal relationships and an enhanced appreciation of life. Although this brief Afterword has focused on the many problems that can occur during hospice care, we must also mention the numerous benefits that are often overlooked.

Patients and families often give indications of gratitude for the care they have received. A friend of mine who spent his final months on a hospital bed in his living room listening to *La Bohème* confided that the final months had been the best time of his long marriage. An 84-year-old woman dying of cancer told me on the last day of her life, 'Dying, you know—is the experience of a lifetime.' A 10-year-old boy whom I knew was cared for at home by his mother and the hospice home care team. On the day he died, when his mother asked him what he wanted for breakfast, he replied, simply, 'A kiss.'

Index